W9-DAX-261

# A
# TREATISE
## ON
# MADNESS.

A

# TREATISE

## ON

# MADNESS.

## By WILLIAM BATTIE M. D.

Fellow of the College of Phyſicians in LONDON,

And Phyſician to St. Luke's Hoſpital.

INTRODUCTION BY
JAMES A. BRUSSEL, M.D., F.A.P.A., F.A.C.P.

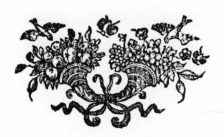

BRUNNER/MAZEL *Publishers* • New York • 1969

Copyright © 1969 by Brunner/Mazel, Inc.
80 East 11th Street, New York, N.Y. 10003
Library of Congress Catalog Card Number 68-56287
Manufactured in the United States of America

# INTRODUCTION

The delight of medical historians is to unearth "firsts"—the first time a hypodermic needle was used, the first case of arthritis reported, and so on. Sometimes a first is not discovered until the one to whom the honor belongs is dead. Such is the case with Dr. William A. Battie, who lived in England from 1704 to 1776. He, his medical accomplishments, and this book form a remarkable series of firsts.

To begin with, Battie was the first teacher of psychiatry in England; some authorities go so far as to say "in the world." Moreover he was more than a rebel who differed with and defied accepted mid-18th century psychiatric thinking—especially as pontificated by John Monro, the director of Bethlehem. He was a pioneer in mental dynamics, in hospital care of the insane, and in the writing of the first extensive book on psychiatry in England. He abhorred the unwholesome conditions at Bethlehem and this led him to be one of the founders of St. Lukes' Hospital for Lunaticks in London where he was superintendent until he left to head a large private asylum.

Battie's *Treatise on Madness* is an especially important work in medical history because it is *"the first by a psychiatrist who could draw on his experiences with a large number of patients . . ."* (Hunter and MacAlpine, *300 Years of Psychiatry*).

As the first psychiatrist to teach his specialty, Battie invites—nay, implores—physicians to read his book, to study psychiatry, to visit his institution (the first private one, incidentally, devoted exclusively to the care and treatment of the insane), to accompany him on rounds, and to make their own observations. This was the more novel because the students were not bound by the centuries-old tradition which prevailed in Bethlehem and which was gospel for the profession.

Besides being a psychiatric first, *A Treatise on Madness* contains some revolutionary (for that time) ideas, many of which are valid by

V

today's criteria. At least Battie sponsored "change"; to throw off the yoke of antiquated and unproven isms and give thought to new concepts even if they turn out to be wrong when given a clinical try-out. Today we call this research. When one reads this book and appreciates how "modern" Battie's medical reasoning is, it is understandable that he would be a minority of one among his contemporary colleagues who, a dozen years after Battie's death, advocated drastic purging, blistering of the skull, bleeding, induction of vomiting, and other similar measures for George III in his first attack of insanity in 1788. Certainly he treated his patients, both at St. Luke's and at his own private hospital, more humanely than did Monro at Bethlehem.

Among his tenets, many of them "firsts," are his (correct) antipathy for violent purging as treatment of the insane. He separates each psychiatric symptom, and maintains that a definition must say what madness is and is not. (Ask any contemporary psychiatrist to define "psychosis" and watch his embarrassment!). He points out that defective sensation is not necessarily psychopathological, differentiates between altered sensation in the normal, the somatically sick, and the insane (to whom he correctly lends the word "delusion" to the perversion or other change in sensation). He envisions sensory pathways and fibers dividing and re-dividing "beyond human vision." Considering his era, Dr. Battie reveals an astounding knowledge of neuro-anatomy. He wipes out the then current misconception that the brain is a gland whose secretion makes sensation possible. He recognizes exogenous and endogenous sources of sensation. Amazingly, he preceded Freud by claiming that all sensation is, at first, crudely received and interpreted by the brain as either painful or pleasurable; this is a faculty necessary "to preserve life." He points out that if an animal holds its breath, anxiety (pain) compels him to exhale. "Uneasy sensation leads to sickness"—certainly a clear description of what we know as psychosomaticism.

He says that madness begins with "too active sensation" and ends with "too languid sensation." Again, in madness, sensation is often disproportional to the external stimulus (today's "over-valuation"). An

VI

unpleasant "external object" may disrupt "natural sensation"; so may "nerve weakness." (And Freud, W. W. Keen and others are credited as pioneers in neurasthenia!). Precipitating causes of madness are "black November days, unpleasant weather" and the "tempest of love, hate, and other passions." Where protracted disease and pains persist, a reactive depression may lead to suicide. Dr. Battie certainly proved that there is nothing new in psychiatry.

There are many more "firsts" in this superb book. It is extremely interesting and should be a reading reward for all who peruse it.

JAMES A. BRUSSEL, M.D., F.A.C.P., F.A.P.A.
*Assistant Commissioner, N. Y. State Department
of Mental Hygiene
Director, Bureau of Historical Research*

*New York, November 1968*

# A
# TREATISE
## ON
# MADNESS.

## By WILLIAM BATTIE M. D.

Fellow of the College of Physicians in LONDON,

And Physician to St. Luke's Hospital.

LONDON:

Printed for J. WHISTON, and B. WHITE, in Fleet-street.

M,DCC,LVIII.

[Price Two Shillings and Six-Pence.]

T O

THE MOST NOBLE

G E O R G E,

Earl of CARDIGAN,

Prefident of ST. LUKE'S HOSPITAL,

THIS

TREATISE ON MADNESS

IS HUMBLY DEDICATED

BY

HIS LORDSHIP's

DUTIFUL AND OBLIGED SERVANT

W. BATTIE.

—————————

# ADVERTISEMENT.

AMONG the many good reafons offered to the Publick, for eſtabliſhing another Hoſpital for the reception of Lunatics, one, and that not the leaſt conſiderable, was *the introducing more Gentlemen of the Faculty to the Study and Practice of one of the moſt important branches of Phyſick.*

The attention of thoſe worthy citizens of *London*, who firſt planned and promoted this charitable work, was carried beyond its more immediate object. Not content with giving relief to a few indigent perſons of their own age or country they intereſted themſelves in the care of poſterity; and as far as they

were

were able made a more ample and effectual provifion for that help, which all Lunatics of whatever nation or quality muft at all times ftand moft in need of.

Agreeably to this their extenfive benevolence, they very foon by an unanimous vote fignified their inclination of admitting young Phyficians well recommended to vifit with me in the Hofpital, and freely to obferve the treatment of the patients there confined.

A command fo conformable to my own fentiments I not only moft readily obeyed; but, that I might anfwer their expectations in this as well as in every other particular to the utmoft of my power, I moreover offered to the perufal of the Gentlemen who honoured me with their attendance the reafons of thofe prefcriptions, which were fubmitted to their obfervation.

The

The end propofed in committing my thoughts to writing on this fubject has induced me to publifh. Thofe, for whofe ufe thefe papers were originally defigned, having encouraged me to hope that the fame hints may be of fervice to other Students, who have not the fame opportunity of feeing practice.

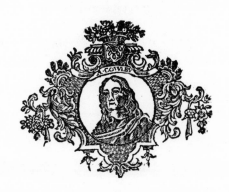

*Lately Published,*

*By* JOHN WHISTON *and* BENJ. WHITE, *in* ONE VOLUME
Quarto, *Price* 12*s. Bound,*

DE PRINCIPIIS ANIMALIBUS Exercitationes viginti quatuor in
Theatro Collegii Medicorum Londinensium habitæ.

## *A* GULIELMO BATTIE, *M.D.*

Collegii ejusdem Socio.

————*Nunquam aliud Natura aliud Sapientia dicit.*

# A

# TREATISE

## ON

# MADNESS.

## SECT. I.

### *The Definition of Madneſs.*

MADNESS, though a terrible and at preſent a very frequent calamity, is perhaps as little underſtood as any that ever afflicted mankind. The names alone uſually given to this diſorder and its ſeveral ſpecies, *viz. Lunacy, Spleen, Melancholy, Hurry of the Spirits, &c.* may convince any one of the

B                                                    truth

truth of this affertion, without having recourfe to the authors who have profeffedly treated on this fubject.

Our defect of knowledge in this matter is, I am afraid, in a great meafure owing to a defect of proper communication: and the difficulties attending the care of Lunaticks have been at leaft perpetuated by their being entrufted to Empiricks, or at beft to a few felect Phyficians, moft of whom thought it advifeable to keep the cafes as well as the patients to themfelves. By which means it has unavoidably happened that in this inftance experience, the parent of medical fcience, has profited little, and every Practitioner at his firft engaging in the cure of Lunacy has had nothing but his own natural fenfe and fagacity to truft to ; except what he may perchance have heard of Antimonial vomits, ftrong purges, and Hellebore, as fpecifically antimaniacal: Which traditional knowledge however, if indifcriminately reduced to practice, a little experience will foon make him wifh he had been an entire ftranger to.

There is therefore reafon to hope, that an attempt to difcover the caufes, effects, and cure of Madnefs, will meet with a favourable reception ; fince, whatever may be the event, the intention

is

is right; and it is some comfort to think that nothing of this nature, even though it should fall
short of what is aimed at, can in its consequences be entirely useless. For the judicious
reader will at least be hereby inclined to turn
his thoughts to the same subject, and may even
receive instruction from the miscarriages of such
an undertaking.

But the peculiar misfortune just now mentioned, *viz.* want of proper communication, though
the chief, is not the only hindrance to our knowledge: for Madness hath moreover shared the
fate common to many other distempers of not
being precisely defined. Inasmuch as not only
several symptoms, which frequently and acciden-
tally accompany it, have been taken into the account as constant, necessary, and essential; but
also the supposed cause, which perhaps never ex-
isted or certainly never acted with such effect,
has been implied in the very names usually given
to this distemper. No wonder therefore is it,
whilst several disorders, really independent of
Madness and of one another, are thus blended
together in our bewildered imagination, that a
treatment, rationally indicated by any of those
disorders, should be injudiciously directed against
Madness itself, whether attended with such symptoms or not. Much less can we blame the Phy-

fician,

fician, who being prejudiced by the fuppofed caufe couched in the name of the diftemper he has to deal with at every new or full Moon attenuates, evacuates, or alters the peccant humours by medicines peculiarly adapted to the black or fplendid Bile, &c.

In order therefore to avoid this mifchievous confufion of fentiment as well as language, and that we may fix a clear and determinate meaning to the Word *Madnefs*; we muft for fome time at leaft quit the fchools of Philofophy, and content ourfelves with a vulgar apprehenfion of things; we muft reject not only every fuppofed caufe of Madnefs, but alfo every fymptom which does not neceffarily belong to it, and retain no one phœnomenon but what is effential, that is without which the word *Madnefs* becomes nugatory and conveys no idea whatever : or, in other words, no definition of Madnefs can be fafe, which does not, with regard at leaft to fome particular fymptoms, determine what it is not, as well as what it is.

Firft then, though too great and too lively a perception of objects that really exift creates an uneafinefs not felt by the generality of men, and therefore difcovers a præternatural ftate in the inftruments of Senfation, and tho' fuch uneafinefs frequently accompanies Madnefs, and is therefore

fore fometimes miftaken for it; neverthelefs Anxiety is no more effentially annexed to Madnefs,
fo as to make part of our complex idea, than
Fever, Head-ach, Gout, or Leprofy. Witnefs the
many inftances of happy Mad-men, who are
perfectly eafy under what is efteemed by every
one but themfelves the greateft misfortune human nature is liable to.

Secondly, though too little and too languid a
perception of things that really exift and are ob-
truded with force fufficient to excite fenfation in
the generality of men, difcovers as præternatural
a ftate or diforder in the inftruments of Senfation
as uncommon Anxiety, and tho' it fometimes attends Madnefs, and is likewife miftaken for it,
efpecially by the *French* who call Mad-men and
Fools by the fame name; neverthelefs fuch defect
of Senfation is no more effentially annexed to
Madnefs than the former fymptom of Anxiety,
which that very frequent fymptom of Madnefs
fufficiently proves.

But--*qui fpecies alias veris capiet, commotus habe-
bitur* --- And this by all mankind as well as the
Phyfician : no one ever doubting whether the
perception of objects not really exifting or not
really correfponding to the fenfes be a certain
fign of Madnefs. Therefore *deluded imagination,*
which

which is not only an indifputable but an effential
character of Madnefs, (that is without which, all
accidental fymptoms being removed from our
thoughts, we have no idea whatever remaining
annexed to that found) precifely difcriminates
this from all other animal diforders: or that man
and that man alone is properly mad, who is fully
and unalterably perfuaded of the Exiftence or of
the appearance of any thing, which either does
not exift or does not actually appear to him, and
who behaves according to fuch erroneous per-
fuafion.

Madnefs, or falfe perception, being then a
præternatural ftate or diforder of Senfation; before we attempt to difcover its caufes effects and
cure, it will be neceffary for us to inveftigate the
feat the caufes and the effects of natural Senfation. For the confideration of the abufe or fault
of any thing neceffarily brings that very thing
into comparifon with what it was when found
and perfect; and 'tis impoffible for us rationally
to amend or reftore what never was the object of
our thoughts.

Be it therefore our firft endeavour to contem-
plate natural Senfation: if haply this moft diftinguifhing property of animal life may fupply us
with actual and pofitive knowledge of fome mat-

ters

ters that relate to the prefent fubject ; or at leaft may point out to us what it is that herein fur-paffes our imperfect underftandings. A fcience negative indeed, and by no means fo fatisfactory to the pride and fpeculative curiofity of man as the former, but very often as ufeful and as con-ducive to the attaining practical truth.

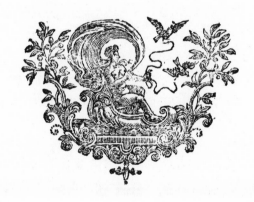

SECT.

## S E C T.  II.

### *The Seat of natural Senfation.*

Whoever is confcious that he hears, fees, or feels, and beholds all animals he is converfant with acting juft in the fame manner as he does when he hears, fees, or feels, muft acknowledge that his own and every other animal body is as really endued with Senfation as that it exifts.

Whoever attentively contemplates in what manner he and every other animal is affected by external impulfe, muft acknowledge that fome parts of the fame body, however animated, are quite infenfible, fome endued with a lefs degree of Senfation than others.

Whoever is moreover fufficiently verfed in Anatomical refearches, and has learnt to feparate thofe parts of an animal body, which, however contiguous or clofely connected, are neverthelefs really diftinct from each other, very readily difcovers feveral foft fibres, each of which is actually divifible into many fmaller of the fame kind, as far as his eye can trace; and he by analogy juftly concludes that each of thofe fmaller fibres

is

is as capable of being ftill farther and farther divided beyond the reach of vifion, and even of human imagination.

Thefe foft fibres are all connected with the contents of the cranium, and in different parts of the body they are collected into fafciculi ; every one of which is enveloped by a continuation of thofe very membranes which within the cranium contain the fubftance of the brain and its medullary appendages.

Every fuch fafciculus as well as the feveral fibres it is refolveable into is called *a Nerve :* a name borrowed indeed from the ancients, but ufed by them in a very different fignification. For by νεῦρον and *nervus* neither the *Greeks* nor *Latins* meant any thing foft and medullary, but on the contrary the hard and elaftic fubftance of a tendon or ligament ; as the word ἀπονεύρωσις, ftill retained by the moderns to fignify the fafcia or membrane expanded over and connecting the mufcular fibres, fufficiently fhews.

Every nerve, which is within the reach of our obfervation, is extended between the *medulla oblongata* or its appendage the *medulla fpinalis* and the place of fuch nerve's deftination. But every fuch nerve is thus extended in a man-

C

ner

ner very different from the difpofition of the
blood-veffels, and indeed of all other portions of
the fame body which are called fimilar.  For
in its paffage it neither is fplit into ramifications,
nor is it at all connected with any contiguous
parts of the body,  except with fome fubftances
equally nervous called ganglions chiefly obfer-
vable in the mefentery.

If a nerve in a living body be diftracted by
external force,  there immediately arifes an exquifite fenfation called pain.   Which fenfation is
always in a direct proportion to the quantity of
fuch diftracting force ;  and which  never  ceafes
either untill the diftracting force is removed or
is become unactive, or untill the material particles which conftitute the faid nerve are by this
diftraction irrecoverably difunited.

If to a nerve in a living body be applied any
acrimonious objects, that is fuch portions of matter whofe furfaces are full of angles,  and which
when affifted with proper impulfe are therefore
capable of diftracting the particles that conftitute
the nervous fubftance,  there immediately arifes
the fame painful fenfation :  which is always in
a direct proportion to the quantity and acutenefs
of fuch acrimonious angles, and to the impulfe
with which they are impacted,  and which continues

tinues as long as in the former cafe of vifible diftraction occafioned by external force.

Thofe parts of an animal body, in which the greateft quantity of nervous fibres is manifeftly contained, and in which fuch nervous fibres lie the moft expofed and undefended by any other matter that conftitutes the fame body, are the fooneft and the moft affected whenever any external objects are applied with force fufficient to excite fenfation.

Thofe membranes, which not only within the cranium furround the brain, but which alfo ferve as fheaths to the feveral appendages of the brain, collecting them into nervous fafciculi all over the body as far as the eye can trace, are indeed every where contiguous to and feem intimately connected with the medullary fubftance they contain: neverthelefs upon the application of any external objects they all difcover no extraordinary figns of fenfibility, any more than feveral other membranes in the fame body, which are equally vafcular and elaftic. Witnefs the many well attefted cafes of erofions and other accidents of the dura mater unattended with any degree of pain.

All

All which conftant and uncontroverted ob-
fervations prove, 1. That the nervous or medullary fubftance derived from or rather communicating with the brain is the feat or inftrument of natural Senfation : 2. That no other
matter whatever, whether animated or not, is
fuch feat or inftrument.

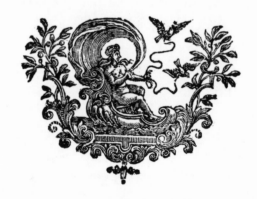

SECT.

## S E C T.  III.

*The supposed Causes of natural Sensation.*

THAT the medullary or nervous substance continued from or rather connected with the brain is the seat of Sensation, is a point now so universally agreed upon,
that perhaps it might have been sufficient barely
to have asserted it without any formal proof.
Happy should we be, if the causes of Sensation
were as clearly and incontestably settled.

But I am afraid before any right or satisfactory
notion can be formed concerning this matter,
we must get rid of some opinions, which however absurd have of late passed upon many for
real knowledge.

The reason of this difference, which at present subsists between the discovery of the seat,
and the discovery of the causes of Sensation, is
not in the things themselves that have been en-
quired after, but in the manner of enquiry.
Because in fixing the seat of Sensation we have
been content with facts that are apparent to all
men, and which if any one should controvert,
he must disclaim the evidence of his own senses:
But

But in affigning the caufes of Senfation feveral things have been affumed as matters of fact, which have never been difcovered, and which may at leaft with equal probability be denied as admitted.

For here the Hypothetical Genius, forgetful that he hath Nature's works for his contemplation, and defpifing that poor pittance of knowledge which the real appearance of things fupplies every one with as well as himfelf, hath dared without any warrant to coin new ideas; hath made free with air, water, æther, nay even electrical fire; and imagining that to be probable which is barely poffible, and then heightening this affumed probability up to matter of fact, he takes one large ftride more and roundly afferts that *the brain is a gland; that its cortical portion is a convolution of fecretory veffels defigned to feparate from the blood one or other of thofe elementary fubftances, which he hath by ways unknown introduced into the carotid arteries for this his prefent purpofe; that the medullary portion of the brain and nerves is nothing elfe but a collection of excretory ducts ferving to convey this elementary matter to all the fenfible parts of the body: which matter either by undulation or retrograde motion imparts to the Senforium commune all thofe impulfes it receives from fuch external objects as*

*affect*

*affect the extremities of the nervous filaments.*
This excrement therefore of the brain tho' in-
vifible is the neceffary caufe of fight, tho' im-
palpable the fufficient caufe of feeling, and
tho' an animal Spirit the material caufe of animal Senfation.

Now, as the fecretion of fuch a nervous fluid
and confequently its very exiftence depends entirely upon the analogy that is fuppofed to lie
between the brain and every glandular fubftance,
in cafe the brain is very unlike a gland in any
material circumftance, this whole machinery is
immediately deftroyed.

Admitting therefore, what has never yet been
proved, that the cortical portion of the brain refembles the fecretory organ of a gland, yet the
medullary or nervous fubftance is different from
all excretory ducts whatever: inafmuch as no excretory duct is ever found but what is immediately detached from the gland whence it iffues ;
whereas on the contrary the fuppofed glandular
or fecretory fubftance of the brain is continued
to every part fupplied with nerves, and thefe
nerves the fuppofed excretory ducts, after that
they have left the cranium and their glandular
origin the brain, wherever they are capable of
being examined, remain as clofely connected

not

not only with the cortical or fecretory portion of the brain, but even with the productions of the dura and pia mater, as the medullary fubftance itfelf whilft contained within the cranium.

This obfervation alone would be fufficient to deftroy the very foundation of a nervous fluid, if any Hypothefis whatever could deferve a ferious confideration. But it may be feared that a folemn confutation of chimæras will appear equally ridiculous as an attempt to eftablifh them; and he may perhaps incur the fufpicion of infanity which thefe theorifts have deferved, who fhall fight in earneft with fhadows, and mifpend his time in offering reafons, why the folid conftituent parts of the medullary fubftance contained in every nerve bid fairer for fupplying us with the material caufe of Senfation, than a fluid never yet difcovered, and which its very authors confefs was once foreign to the body, and even extracted from dead and putrefcent matter fpirited up, we know not how, into animality.

Let us therefore quit this enchanted ground to thofe, if fuch there be, who are ftill inclined to difpute upon it; and in order to clear our way a little more to the real caufes of Senfation, let us divert our attention to a very common phrafe, *viz. weaknefs of nerves,* which tho' not profeffedly

feffedly fyftematical, like the former fcheme of *animal fpirits*, is neverthelefs extremely delufive ; inafmuch as it feems indirectly to offer another folution of the phœnomenon in queftion, and to afcertain the caufe of Senfation.

For fince the word *weaknefs*, when joined with material fubftances, can convey no idea but a lax cohæfion of fuch particles as conftitute thofe fubftances ; therefore the phrafe *weaknefs of nerves*, which denotes a morbid excefs of Senfation, feems to imply that Senfation itfelf is owing to the loofe cohæfion of thofe material particles which conftitute the nervous fubftance, inafmuch as the quantity of every effect muft be proportionable to its caufe.

By this inaccurate manner of talking, the moft diftinguifhing property of animal nature is in danger of being blended with inanimate matter. For, if the cafe really were what thefe words feem to import, all bodies whofe particles do not cohære with too great a degree of proximity would be nervous, that is endued with Senfation. But, fince no portion of matter, however loofely compacted, is nervous except it is part of an animal body, therefore the medullary fubftance of a nerve is endued with Senfation not becaufe its conftituent particles are loofely united :

D                                                and

and every nervous filament, tho' it confifts of parts extended and not too clofely cohæring, is confeffedly as diftinct from every other material fubftance confifting of parts extended and equally cohæring, as a man from a carcas, or an horfe from an equeftrian ftatue.

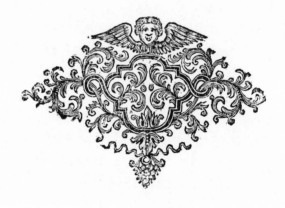

SECT.

## S E C T.  IV.

*The real Causes of natural Senfation.*

SENSATION, however perplexed it may feem to thofe who too curioufly enquire into its nature, is to the modeft obferver as clear in idea and as fully to be accounted for, at leaft to all ufeful intents and purpofes, as any phœnomenon whatever.

For is not what we feel a plain matter of fact, of which we are not only certain and confcious ourfelves, but which we are likewife capable of communicating to others by words or figns? And are we not perfectly well acquainted with many things, which when impelled with force fufficient will make us feel; and which it is frequently in our power to apply, remove, or avoid, as beft fuits our intereft?

It is the heedlefs or rather the wilful neglect of precifely feparating thefe many evident and external caufes of Senfation as well from their unknown and internal operations as from their in-termediate and equally unknown effects, that has created fuch difficulties in contemplating this phœnomenon.

For

For the mutual cohæsion of material particles, as effential to our idea of an animal body as fenfe itfelf, but not better accounted for, hath however been looked upon as a thing much lefs myfterious.

Which feeming diverfity can be owing to no-thing elfe, but becaufe the generality of man-kind have contented themfelves with the ufeful and the attainable knowledge of fuch external objects, as will harden or foften thofe bodies they are applied to, without enquiring too nice-ly why the conftituent particles of thofe bodies are more or lefs united upon fuch application, or indeed why they are united at all : whereas the philofopher in his contemplation of fenfible matter is not content with knowing certainly like other men what objects externally applied to a nerve will create, increafe, or deaden fenfation, but moreover conjectures why ; and attempts by any means whatever to affign the manner in which thefe external objects act upon, and the changes they produce in the nervous fubftance previous to fenfation their laft effect ; which ef-fect, for reafons beft known to himfelf, feems to demand a more explicit folution than the co-hæfion of material particles.

In.

In endeavouring therefore to affign the caufes of Senfation, be it one of our chiefeft cares to diftinguifh them from one another as effectually in our mind, as they are really different in their nature, and to feparate what we actually and ufefully know from what we are, and perhaps fhall always be without any great damage, entirely ignorant of.

For which purpofe, it may not be amifs to premife a few confiderations on caufes in general; which will illuftrate the fubject of our prefent enquiry and at the fame time be confirmed thereby.

Firft then, by obferving that any one phœnomenon frequently follows another, we conclude that the fecond is owing to the firft; and hence we get the ideas of *caufe* and *effect*.

Secondly, by obferving that any one phœnomenon never fails to follow another, we conclude that the firft is not only a caufe but alfo a fufficient caufe of the fecond.

Thirdly, by obferving that the fecond phœnomenon never occurs but in confequence of the firft, we further conclude that the firft is not
only

only a caufe but a neceffary caufe of the fecond, which is therefore called the *caufa fine qua non.*

Fourthly, by obferving that the fecond phœnomenon follows the firft without either the evident or the demonftrated intervention of any other phœnomenon as neceffary or at leaft acceffary to its exiftence, we conclude that the firft phœnomenon is moreover the immediate caufe of the fecond.

Fifthly, by obferving either that the firft phœnomenon is not always fucceeded by the fecond, or that the fecond is not always preceded by the firft, we conclude that the firft phœnomenon is either not a fufficient or not a neceffary, but merely an accidental caufe of the fecond.

Sixthly, by obferving or by admitting as undeniable that any one or more phœnomena intervene between the firft and the laft in queftion, we plainly difcover that the firft is remote, and that the feveral other intervening phœnomena in their order approach nearer and nearer to the immediate caufe.

Seventhly, a very little reflection upon caufes and effects as thus ftated will make us conclude that the remote and accidental caufes of any
effect

effect may be many, but that the fufficient and neceffary as well as the immediate caufe can be but one. Since either of two caufes fuppofed fufficient will render the other unneceffary ; and either caufe fuppofed neceffary will render the other infufficient. Which unavoidable conclu-fion, by the way, might be extended beyond fecondary agents or inftruments, improperly cal-led caufes, and would give an additional proof, if any was wanting, to the unity of the firft, the neceffary, the fufficient, and indeed ftrictly fpeaking the fole caufe of all things.

Thus, to inftance in our prefent fubject ; fight, hearing, tafte, fmell, &c. which frequently fuc-ceed the application of external objects, are look-ed upon by us as the effects of fuch external ob-jects ; and we in common difcourfe refer our ideas back to thofe objects as to their caufes, as when we fay *we fee the fun, we hear the drum, &c.*

But, forafmuch as the external objects of fenfe, however forcible their application may be, do not always and in all animal bodies create fight, &c. And moreover, as the very fame perceptions do fometimes, at leaft in difordered fubjects, arife without any external object that really affects them ; it is impoffible but every fuch external object muft be meerly accidental, and by no

means

means the fufficient or the neceffary caufe of
fuch its nervous effect : Which fufficient and neceffary caufe is therefore internal, that is it in-
hæres in the very frame and conftitution of the
nervous fubftance itfelf; whereby alone fuch
fubftance is rendered capable of being affected
by any external object fo as to create Senfation ;
and without which internal caufe no thing whatever would actually become an object of our
fenfes.

For the fame reafon all fuch external caufes
are not only accidental but likewife remote.
Since the neceffary and fufficient caufe at leaft
muft intervene ; and befides, before an external
object can create any fenfation whatever, it
muft produce feveral intermediate effects, *viz.*
motion, impulfe, and preffure : all which precede not only fight, *&c.* thereby excited, but
alfo precede that particular internal affection of
the nerve itfelf, whatever it is, which is the immediate, the neceffary, and the fufficient caufe
of fuch perception.

The accidental and remote caufes of Senfation, as alfo their intermediate effects, provided
fuch effects are external to the nervous fubftance, very readily difcover themfelves, and are
clearly comprehended. For indeed they are all
bodies

bodies that lye within our obſervation (many of which are within our reach) and the motion and impulſe of thoſe bodies, or of particles emitted therefrom, upon the organs of ſenſe : which every one not only has a clear idea of, but is moreover certain of their exiſtence, motion, and impulſe.

Now, as no body whatever can be capable of creating Senſation in conſequence of its motion and impulſe, without preſſing upon the nerve affected by ſuch impulſe ; therefore preſſure of the medullary ſubſtance contained in the nervous filaments approaches nearer in order to the immediate cauſe of Senſation, than the motion and impulſe of any external object.

Preſſure of the medullary ſubſtance contained in the nervous filaments cannot indeed be imagined without ſome alteration in the former arrangement of thoſe material particles which conſtitute that ſubſtance. But we have no idea whatever, either viſible or intellectual, how and in what manner thoſe particles are by ſuch preſſure differently juxtapoſited, previouſly to Senſation thereby excited.

Whence it undeniably follows that preſſure upon the medullary ſubſtance contained in the

E                              nervous

nervous filaments is the laſt in order of all thoſe cauſes of Senſation, which we have any idea of. Thus far and no farther our knowledge in theſe matters reaches, limited by the outſide of the ſeat of Senſation ; what paſſes within being meer conjecture. For if a new poſition of medullary particles, which is an immediate and unavoidable effect of external preſſure, does not diſcover it-ſelf any more than their conſtitutional arrange-ment ; what account can we with any the leaſt degree of modeſty pretend to give of all the alterations in the nervous ſubſtance ſtill ſubſe-quent to ſuch preſſure and to change of place thereby occaſioned ; a regular ſeries of which may, for any thing we know to the contrary, precede the immediate cauſe of ſenſation.

SECT.

## SECT. V.

*The salutary Effects of natural Sensation.*

SENSATION is always accompanied with some degree of pleasure or uneasiness ; no animal being indifferent to what he sees, hears, or feels. These additional and in some degree inseparable affections demonstrate the direct tendency of Sensation to the preservation of life ; inasmuch as every one spontaneously flies from those objects which hurt and are at enmity with him, and covets such as create satisfaction and are suitable to his interest.

But, tho' no one at first sight would doubt whether the perception of pleasure is agreeable to his nature, and conducive to its preservation ; it may with great reason be doubted by those who reflect a little whether such perception, however convenient it may seem to animal life, is alone instrumental in its preservation, and without the intervention of the contrary affection ever conduces to health.

For uneasiness is so interwoven in the very frame of mortals, that even the greatest present

satis-

satisfaction implies the removing or stifling the greatest uneasiness which before disquieted. And a sense of future pleasure, as it excites desire, in that very desire implies a present uneasiness adequate to the supposed enjoyment of the pleasure in expectation. By which present uneasiness, according to Mr. *Locke*'s just observation, the will is determined.

However paradoxical therefore it may seem, nothing is more true than that Anxiety, a real evil, is nevertheless productive of real good; and, tho' seemingly disagreeable to Nature, is absolutely necessary to our preservation, in such a manner, that without its severe but useful admonitions the several species of animals would speedily be destroyed.

For first, are not hunger and thirst very salutary Anxieties? By which the nerves of the mouth œsophagus and stomach excite all animals from the first moment of their birth to seize on such objects, as are capable of relieving those natural and healthy but agonizing sensations.

Now the real good produced by the gratification of these appetites is by no means to be placed in their present gratification alone. Whatever he may imagine, who being ignorant of the

animal

animal œconomy looks no farther than the actual pleaſure which accompanies the ſtifling ſuch ſenſations. For the end herein propoſed by the Author of Nature is undoubtedly the refection of that very body which hungers and thirſts; whoſe conſtituent particles by the inevitable effects of vital action are in a continual flux and decay; whereas the efficient or coercive cauſes of eating and drinking are thoſe ſenſations alone, which torment every animal to a very good purpoſe. Who perhaps would not otherwiſe give himſelf the trouble of opening his mouth, much leſs by hard labour earn food wherewith to fill it; even tho' he ſhould be aſſured that the loſs of meat and drink to-day, tho' not at all inconvenient to him at preſent, will be ſenſibly felt to-morrow by his diſtempered body, and that his idleneſs and faſting will be ſoon attended by fatal conſequences.

Secondly, the introducing freſh air into the lungs being as neceſſary for the immediate continuance of life, as it is for other purpoſes of the animal œconomy which are more remote, and at preſent unknown; therefore every animal provided with organs of reſpiration, whether awake or ſleeping, draws into his breaſt and expels a quantity of external air ſufficient to diſtend them from the firſt moment of his birth

till

till the laft period of life. Which alternate
action, if he either carelefsly or obftinately omits
it, he is very foon compelled to perform by that
inexpreffible Anxiety which attends a long de-
tention of air once admitted as well as the re-
fufing admiffion to any air at all.

Thirdly, forafmuch as voluntary exercife of
the body is no lefs requifite to the due circulation and fecretions of the animal fluids, and the
falutary confequences thereon depending, than
the propulfive action of the heart and the refilition of the arterial tubes ; which the ill effects
of a fedentary life fufficiently prove ; therefore
the uneafy fenfation that is always occafioned by
fatiety and the wearifome condition of idlenefs
determine all animals, to whom activity is thus
neceffary, frequently to alter their place of refi-
dence, and to remove from thofe objects they
have long been converfant with, however pleafing and eagerly fought for they might once have
been.

Fourthly, all the afore-mentioned inftances
of uneafy fenfation, however nearly allied to
and often ending in ficknefs, are neverthelefs
the natural effects of perfect health. But befides thefe there occur feveral other anxieties,
which are the unavoidable effects of real ficknefs

and

and moreover frequently determine the will of the patient to such things as are capable either of relieving the present disorder or of preventing its mischievous consequences. Thus, to instance in one particular, feaverish heat threatens putrid obstructions, and at the same time occasions intense thirst and an almost insatiable craving for acidulated water. Which desire, if not contradicted by the officious and ill-tim'd care of the by-standers, procures a remedy that is both diluting and antiseptic.

Lastly, tho' the nervous energy be neither absolutely necessary nor alone sufficient to excite muscular action, yet such is the connection between the nervous and muscular fibres, however really distinct from each other, that animal sensation often instantaneously precedes animal action, so as to have confounded these two qualities, or at least to have made the one appear the immediate and only cause of the other. And, what chiefly deserves our notice whilst we are considering the salutary effects of Sensation, Convulsion itself, a distempered excess of animal motion, which is a frequent effect of uneasy Sensation, sometimes becomes its sudden and efficacious remedy, by removing the material cause of such uneasy Sensation, and that without

any

any determination or interpofition of the will whatever.

All which nervous appetites as well as mufcular motions, that either preferve or reftore health, and are feemingly excited by fomewhat rationally forecafting their falutary ends, have given rife, I fuppofe, to fome modern metaphorical expreffions, *viz. Nature,* and the *Anima* invented by *Willis* and deifyed by *Stahl.* Which figurative words, tho' not quite philofophical, are innocent and even ufeful, in cafe they are applied only to avoid periphrafes in relating medical matters of fact. But young Practitioners, who are often told that they are to imitate and affift Nature, muft take great care not to be mifguided by the literal fenfe of words, or fancy any thing like perfonal confcioufnefs and intellectual agency in the animal œconomy. For in fuch cafe of mifapprehenfion thefe and the like expreffions become as abfurd as all the exploded *Faculties of the Ancients,* and, what is much worfe, may be as mifchievous as an inftrument of death in the hands of a Madman.

SECT.

## SECT. VI.

*The Caufes and Effects of Anxiety and Infenfi-
bility, two fpecies of Senfation difordered tho'
not delufive.*

HAVING contemplated the feat caufes
and effects of natural and true Senfation; before we proceed to confider
delufive Senfation, the only fubject of this enquiry, it may be not improper to take fome notice of thofe two other diforders of the fame
quality, which were excluded from our definition
of Madnefs, *viz.* præternatural *Anxiety* or Senfation too greatly excited by real objects, and its
contrary *Infenfibility* or Senfation not fufficiently
excited by real objects, tho' acting with their ufual
force and tho' capable of engaging the attention
of all other healthy animals of the fame fpecies.

For, although Madnefs in its proper fenfe be
clearly diftinct from the too lively or the too languid perception of things really exifting, it however very often is preceded by or accompanied
with the firft and as often terminates in the fecond of thefe two diforders. Befides the being
too much affected by external impulfe, tho' it

F                                        does

does by no means imply Senſation materially deluſive, inaſmuch as the ideas excited by ſuch impulſe are referred to true and correſponding objects; yet the quantity of concomitant affection
not being proportionate and therefore not in all
reſpects correſponding to the natural quantity of
its real cauſe hath apparently ſome deviation from
abſolute truth, and from the natural and uſual
circumſtances of this animal function. And Senſation not proportionate to real impulſe, tho' it
is not ſtrictly ſpeaking deluſive, hath however as
great a deviation from abſolute truth as exceſſive
Senſation itſelf.

Now Senſation, which in its moſt natural and
perfect ſtate is ſooner or later attended with ſome
degree of uneaſineſs, may with very little addi-
tion be heightened into Anxiety either by the too
great or too long continued force of external objects, or by the illconditioned ſtate of the nerve
itſelf, whereby it is rendered liable to be too
much affected with the uſual action of ſuch external objects.

This illconditioned ſtate of the nerve may be
inhærent in the internal proper and unknown
conſtitution of the medullary ſubſtance, or it
may be external to that ſubſtance, and ariſe from
the loſs or defect of thoſe membranes which en-
velope

velope and fheathe the feat of Senfation, and are
defigned to protect it from fuch rude attacks and
impreffions as might otherwife endanger the dif-
folution of fo foft a matter.

For, whenever thofe integuments are quite removed from a nerve which is endued with no
more than a common fhare of fenfibility, Anxiety muft enfue the application of any external
objects that are capable of exciting natural Senfation. And in fact we find that the laying
bare any fenfible part and expofing it to the
common air, which ufually refrefhes the body
whilft cloathed with fkin, immediately diftracts
us with intolerable torment.

For the fame reafon Anxiety, which follows
an entire removal of the nervous fheaths, will in
fome degree arife whenever thofe fheaths are not
ftrong and fufficiently compacted fo as to anfwer
the purpofe of defence. That is the fenfation
of the nervous or medullary fibres, tho' they continue the fame, will be in a reverfe proportion
to the cohæfion of thofe minute particles which
conftitute the folid and elaftic fibres. And in
fact we find that Anxiety is almoft always the
confequence of morbid laxity, except where the
intervention of fat, lymph, or vifcid congeftions

F 2                                             owing

owing to such laxity substitute an occasional defence.

No wonder is it then that the straining or loosening the solid parts of human bodies should frequently render those bodies liable to be violently affected by such objects as are scarce felt or attended to by other men, who enjoy a natural or artificial strength and compactness of fibres.

And from hence we are enabled to annex a true and intelligible meaning to that expression before taken notice of, *viz. weakness of nerves.* Which word *weakness* would not have been so improper, if it had been joined in idea not to that substance which is strictly nervous, but to its integuments and contiguous membranes; and if laxity, an accidental and remote cause of excessive and therefore uneasy Sensation, had not been thereby made liable to be mistaken for its immediate necessary and sufficient cause.

Whatever may be the cause of Anxiety, it chiefly discovers itself by that agonising impatience observable in some men of black *November* days, of easterly winds, of heat, cold, damps, &c. Which real misery of theirs is sometimes derided by duller mortals as a whimsical affectation.
And

And of the fame nature are the perpetual tempefts of love, hatred, and other turbulent paffions provoked by nothing or at moft by very trifles. In which ftate of habitual difeafes many drag on their wretched lives; whilft others, unequal to evils of which they fee no remedy but death, rafhly refolve to end them at any rate. Which very frequent cafes of fuicide, though generally afcribed to Lunacy by the verdict of a good-natured Jury, except where the deceafed hath not left affets, are no more entitled to the benefit of paffing for pardonable acts of madnefs, than he who deliberately has killed the man he hated deferves to be acquitted as not knowing what he did.

Among the morbid effects of Anxiety or the præternatural excefs of Senfation one, which frequently attends upon it and more particularly demands our attention, is Spafm or the præternatural excefs of mufcular action. Which ftate of morbid motion, tho' fometimes falutary as has been before obferved, is oftner occafioned by this nervous diforder to no good purpofe whatever; and, when very violent or of long continuance, is neceffarily productive of numberlefs evils and of acute and chronical diftempers, which if not relieved in time almoft always end in death.

Another

Another effect of Anxiety or of the præternatural excefs of Senfation is the nervous diforder directly contrary to it, *viz.* Infenfibility, that is a præternatural defect or total lofs of Senfation.

Whether this entire change from one extream to the other is owing to the material inftruments of Senfation having been ftrained by Anxiety or rather by fome of its caufes, cannot perhaps be determined with any degree of certainty. But thus much is clear in reafon that any diftraction, which is fufficient to difunite or break in pieces the medullary fubftance, muft be fufficient to make it unfit for its function; and it is as undeniable in fact that Anxiety is frequently either attended with fuch fpafmodic diforders or occafioned by fuch external injuries as muft neceffarily diftract the nerves thereby affected.

Not that Infenfibility is owing to no other caufe except Anxiety. For it is at leaft as often occafioned by the internal and unknown conftitution of the nervous or medullary fubftance itfelf, which was either formed imperfect at firft or hath fince degenerated.

And

And, befides the internal and unknown defect in the feat of Senfation, Infenfibility may as often be afcribed to another caufe external to the nerve and fufficiently underftood. For, fince the nervous integuments or neighbouring membranes do fheathe the medullary fubftance, and thereby prevent the morbid excefs of its energy ; whenever the fibres that compofe thofe integuments or membranes are præternaturally compacted and of too clofe a texture, inftead of moderating they undoubtedly muft deaden or deftroy Senfation. And for the fame reafon thofe nerves that are pillowed with fat, foaked in lymph, or ftifled by obftructed veffels, cannot and in fact do not receive a proper that is a fenfible impulfe from external objects, altho' fuch objects are rightly and forcibly applied, and although the nervous fubftance itfelf is perfectly found, and in its internal conftitution fitted for the efficacious reception of fuch external impulfe.

But, whatever may be the caufe of Infenfibility, its ill effects are many and as obvious as they are unavoidable, and need not be here enumerated. For they are all thofe diforders in the animal œconomy, which Senfation in its natural vigour was defigned to prevent. The

defect

defect therefore or lofs of this falutary and vital quality muft either hurry on or fuffer the fickly body to approach nearer and nearer to the laft period of animal life.

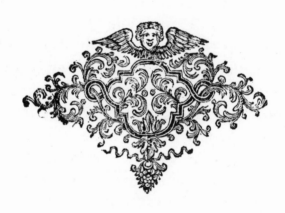

SECT.

## S E C T.   VII.

### *The   Caufes   of   Madnefs.*

WHoever is fatisfied with our account of the feat and caufes of natural and true Senfation, will acknowledge that the one immediate neceffary and fufficient caufe of the præternatural and falfe perception of objects, which either do not exift, or which do not in this inftance excite fuch fenfation, muft be fome diforder of that fubftance which is medullary and ftrictly nervous. And moreover, as he cannot difcover the natural and internal conftitution of this medullary fubftance, which renders it fit for the proper perception of real and external impulfe or rather of the ideas thereby excited; he muft for the fame reafon own that he is unable to difcover wherein confifts that præternatural and internal ftate of the fame nervous matter, which difpofes it to be without any fuch impulfe affected by thofe very ideas, that would have been prefented to the imagination, if the fame nervous matter had been acted upon by fomething external. Or, to fpeak more technically, forafmuch as the one immediate neceffary and fufficient caufe of the perception of real objects

G                                                     is

is unknown, we muſt likewiſe remain entirely ignorant of the one immediate neceſſary and ſufficient cauſe of the perception of Chimæras, which exiſt no where except in the brain of a Madman.

But, altho' the immediate and internal cauſe of deluſive as well as of true Senſation is abſolutely hid, many remoter and external cauſes thereof frequently diſcover themſelves to the by-ſtander, notwithſtanding that the idea thus excited is not by the patient himſelf referred to any one of thoſe true cauſes, but to ſomething elſe, which may or may not exiſt, and which certainly does not in this particular caſe act upon the affected organ.

Thus, to inſtance in a very common accident, the eye that is violently ſtruck immediately ſees flames flaſh before it ; which idea of fire preſented to the imagination plainly ſhews that thoſe material particles which conſtitute the medullary ſubſtance of the optic nerve are affected by ſuch blow exactly in the ſame manner, as they are when real fire acts upon the eye of a man awake and in his ſenſes with force ſufficient to provoke his attention. Thus variety of ſounds diſturb the ear that is ſhocked by the pulſation of veſſels, by the inflammation or other

obſtruction

obstruction of those membranes which line the *meatus auditorius,* by the intrusion of water, and in short by any material force external to the medullary portion of the seventh pair of nerves ; which force hath no connection with any sonorous body, that by its elastic vibration communicates an undulatory motion to the intermediate air.

Now suppose that any one perfectly awake without the accident of such a blow sees fire, or without the pulsation of vessels, inflammation, or any obstruction in the *meatus auditorius, &c.* hears sounds ; or suppose that the idea of flame really excited by a blow is by him referred to an house on fire, or the idea of sound excited by the pulsation of vessels, *&c.* is referred to a musical instrument, which is not near enough to be heard, or is not really played upon ; the man who is so mistaken, and who cannot be set right either upon his own recollection or the information of those about him, is in the apprehension of all sober persons a Lunatic.

From whence we may collect that Madness with respect to its cause is distinguishable into two species. The first is solely owing to an internal disorder of the nervous substance : the second is likewise owing to the same nervous substance be-

G 2                                                    ing

ing indeed in like manner difordered, but difordered *ab extra*; and therefore is chiefly to be attributed to fome remote and accidental caufe. The firft fpecies, until a better name can be found, may be called *Original*, the fecond may be called *Confequential Madnefs*.

The internal diforder of the medullary fubftance, or the caufe of Original Madnefs, for the fame reafon as the immediate neceffary and fufficient caufe of true Senfation, can be but one: but the external and accidental caufes of Confequential Madnefs, as well as of true Senfation, may be many.

Now no external caufe whatever can be fuppofed capable of exciting delufive any more than true perception, except fuch caufe acts materially upon the nerve thereby difordered, and that with force fufficient to alter the former arrangement of its medullary particles. Which force neceffarily implies impulfe and preffure in delufive Senfation, in the fame manner and order as it does in the perception of objects really correfponding thereto.

Preffure therefore amongft all the external and difcoverable caufes of falfe as well as of true perception is in our apprehenfion the neareft to fuch its apparent effect. As to the intermediate alterations

terations of the medullary fubftance, that may really precede delufive Senfation, they are all as much unknown as are the nervous effects which intervene between the preffure made by any external object and the true and adequate idea of that very object.

But, altho' Confequential Madnefs cannot be fuppofed without fome fort and degree of preffure upon the nerves, neverthelefs every fort and degree of preffure does not always and unavoidably produce Confequential Madnefs. For the nerves may fuffer external impulfe, and yet the preffure thereby occafioned either may not have force fufficient to excite any idea at all; or it may act with too great a force and in fo fhocking a manner as to diffolve or greatly difunite the medullary matter; in which cafe Senfation, which can never exift but whilft that matter does properly cohere, inftead of being perverted will be abolifhed, or at leaft fufpended untill the conftituent particles are reunited.

What this particular fort and degree of preffure is, which is capable of creating delufive Senfation, we are not able to afcertain; becaufe the different circumftances of the unknown fubject acted upon will make the nervous effects variable and oftentimes contrary, notwithftanding the action

tion of the known caufe confidered *per fe* is in all refpects the fame.

But, altho' we cannot exactly defcribe the particular ftrength of that external impulfe which excites, any more than we can difcover why it excites delufive ideas ; thus much we may rea-fonably conclude in general that all material ob-jects, which by their action or refiftance occa-fion a fufficient but not too great a preffure upon the medullary fubftance contained in the nerves, may be the remoter caufes of Confequential Mad-nefs.

Which conclufion is not only agreeable to reafon, but is moreover confirmed by matter of fact and almoft every day's experience. Witnefs the internal exoftofes of the cranium, the indu-rations of the finus's and proceffes of the Dura Mater, which have frequently been found in thofe who died mad ; witnefs the intrapreffion of the fkull or concuffion of the head, which if not apoplectic is almoft always attended with a delirium. And indeed every one, who contem-plates feveral cafes of Confequential Madnefs and thofe accidents which precede the fame, will find that preffure of the medullary fubftance fomewhere or other collected intervenes between fuch accidents and thefe their delirious effects.

One

One cafe of Confequential Madnefs that proves
the intervention of fuch preffure is an effect of
Infolation or what the *French* call *coup du Soleil.*
An inftance of which I lately met with in a Sai-
lor, who became raving mad in a moment while
the Sun beams darted perpendicularly upon his
head. Which maniacal effect of heat could be
attributed to no affignable caufe, except either to
the violent impreffion of the Sun's rays upon the
medullary fubftance of the brain, which the cranium in this cafe was not able to defend, or to
the intermediate rarefaction of blood contained in
the veffels of the Dura or Pia Mater, which veffels
being fuddenly diftended compreffed the fame
medullary fubftance. Of the fame nature and
owing to the fame rarefaction of fluids in the
brain are thofe delirious fevers called Calentures;
one of which was, I fuppofe, miftaken for the
plague by the * Author of the *Phyficians laft Le-
gacy,* and treated with bleeding *ufque ad animi
deliquium,* which indeed is its only cure.

Another cafe of Confequential Madnefs is a
fudden inflammation arifing in thofe membranes
which furround and therefore when thus diftended comprefs the contents of the cranium and its
nervous appendages. This ftate of inflammation
whilft

* Dr. *Dover,*

whilft the patient lives difcovers itfelf by the fudden rednefs of the eyes external coat, which is
a part or rather a produ&ion of the Dura Mater:
and that membrane after death is frequently upon
diffe&ion found turgid and difcoloured with a
red bloody fuffufion, juft in the fame manner
as if it had been artificially inje&ed.

Another cafe of Confequential Madnefs is a
gradual congeftion of ferum or other fluid matter upon the fame membranes which envelop the
medullary fubftance; whereby thofe membranes,
tho' not with equal danger as when they are fuddenly inflamed, yet with the fame delirious ef-
fe&s comprefs their nervous contents. This ferous congeftion is difcoverable by the opaque and
cloudy appearance of the cornea, for the fame
reafon as an inflammatory tumor in the Dura
Mater is betrayed by the external coat of the eye
being tinged with blood.

Preffure of the medullary fubftance, the neareft in our apprehenfion to Madnefs of all its
known and remoter caufes, moft frequently and
moft effe&ually produces this its nervous effe&,
whilft it a&s upon the contents of the cranium,
as is evident from the cafes above-mentioned.
But, altho' the brain is undoubtedly the princi-
pal feat of delufive fenfation, neverthelefs it is
not

not the only one : forafmuch as the fame fangui-
nary or ferous obftructions are capable in any other
nervous part of the body of exciting falfe ideas as
well as in the brain, at leaft to fome degree and
in proportion to the quantity of medullary matter
there collected fo as to be fufficiently compreffed
by fuch obftructions. Thus the ftomach, inteftines, and uterus, are frequently the real feats of
Madnefs, occafioned by the contents of thefe vif-
cera being ftopt in fuch a manner as to comprefs
the many nervous filaments, which here commu-
nicate with one another by the mefenteric gan-
glia, and which enrich the contents of the abdomen with a more exquifite fenfation. Thus
the glutton who goes to-bed upon a full ftomach
is hagridden in his fleep. Thus

*Men prove with child as powerful fancy works :*

And patients truly hypochondriacal or hyfterical
refer that load of uneafinefs they feel in their
bellies to fome imaginary object, which if it really
exifted and acted upon their fenfes would excite
the very fame idea.

H                    SECT.

## SECT. VIII.

### *The Causes of Madness.*

FOrasmuch as præternatural preſſure upon
the nerves is in human apprehenſion the
neareſt to deluſive ſenſation thereby excited ; whatever injury creates ſuch preſſure muſt
be a remoter cauſe of Conſequential Madneſs.

Under this head therefore of remoter cauſes
are to be ranked the internal exoſtoſes of the
cranium, the induration of the Dura Mater, the
fracture and intropreſſion of the ſkull and concuſſion of the head, as alſo, if it were of any
ſervice in the cure of madneſs to enumerate
them, the many and various accidents theſe delirious injuries may be owing to.

To the ſame number of remoter cauſes we
muſt add morbid diſtenſions of the veſſels contiguous to the medullary ſubſtance. And, as ſeveral caſes mentioned in the foregoing ſection are
clearly reſolvable into ſuch diſtenſions, whoſe removal or diminution will frequently be ſufficient
to anſwer our intention and is almoſt always neceſſary and ſerviceable in the cure of this diſtem-
per ;

per; it may be of ufe to fpend a little time in examining into the nature and origin of thofe vafcular diftenfions which end in Confequential Madnefs.

Whoever has attended to the accidents that animal bodies are liable to muft have obferved that feveral membranes, which in their natural ftate appear fmooth and even, are fometimes fuddenly at other times gradually elevated beyond the furface or plane they before helped, to compofe. To the firft of thefe two cafes writers on Surgery have given the name of *Tumors by Fluxion*, to the fecond that of *Tumors by Congeftion*; thereby afcribing the quick or flow appearance of thefe fwellings to the different motion of the fluids themfelves, which materially formed them, and which according to the medical philofophy then in fafhion contained all the refources of life health and ficknefs.

Now, altho' the difcovery of the blood's circulation hath demonftrated that the fluids are paffive in every circumftance of animal life whether found or diftempered, it will however be very ufeful in profecuting the prefent enquiry to take into our account the cafes themfelves as diftinguifhed from one another by their different manner of appearance which cannot be contro-

verted,

verted, and then endeavour to affign other reafons for fuch their appearance, which not only
really exift, but which alfo are fufficient to produce either fpecies of tumor.

Tumors then by Fluxion ending in Madnefs
are either veffels diftended by the rarefaction of
their proper and natural contents, as in the cafe
of Infolation ; or, which is the moft frequent accident, they are the fame veffels obftructed by
the fudden intrufion of improper fluids into
fmaller canals which were never defigned to give
either a paffage or admittance to fuch contents,
as in the cafe of Inflammation. Now this change
of place and forcible propulfion of fluids from
their natural ducts into improper receptacles muft
apparently be owing to fome power external to
the fluids fo propelled, which power either was
not excited or did not effectually act the moment
before fuch delirious obftructions took place. But
the fpafmodic conftriction of thofe mufcular fibres which furround the extremities of arteries
and veins, and are at reft till ruffled by fome accident, is a power occafionally excited, and
when acting with fufficient force is capable of
driving the blood out of its natural channels into
veffels not originally fitted for its reception. And
it is moreover a repeated obfervation that Madnefs frequently fucceeds or accompanies Fever,
Epilepfy,

Epilepfy, Child-birth, and the like mufcular diforders; and that the tumultuous and vifibly fpafmodic paffions of joy and anger are all at leaft
for a time maniacal. But thefe paffions con-
ftringe the mufcles of the head and neck, and
therefore like a ligature force the blood that was
defcending in the jugular veins back upon the
minuteft veffels of the brain.

Spafm therefore, when it is productive of tumors by Fluxion or of fudden diftenfions in the
veffels contiguous to the nervous fubftance, as alfo
fpafmodic paffions fuch as joy and anger are to
be reckoned amongft the remoter caufes of Madnefs. Not but that the fame mufcular conftriction is often excited by the application of feveral
external objects; which objects are therefore to
be added to the fame clafs. For befides the many well attefted cafes of poifons or medicines,
which as foon as fwallowed convulfe the body
and intoxicate the underftanding, fuch as Hem-
loc, and the root lately miftaken for Gentian,
fuch as Opium when adminiftered to fome particular patients, &c. The many bottle-com-
panions whofe pulfes beat high and quick, whofe
faces are flufhed with blood in the fame manner
as if they were ftrangled, who are firft wild and
then ftupid, who drink till they fee double, and
then drink on till they cannot fee at all, as well

as.

as the crowds of wretches that infeft our ftreets and fill our hofpitals, evidently prove to the vulgar as well as to the Phyfician that vinous fpirits inftantaneoufly provoke an irregular action of the mufcles fucceeded by temporary delirium; and that, if the fame noxious draughts are taken in too large dofes or frequently repeated, they become a very common tho' remoter caufe of continual madnefs.

If any one rather fuppofes that fuch external objects, which produce Madnefs, act immediately upon the nerves thereby affected, and that fpafm, tho' an undoubted effect of the fame objects, is the companion and not the intervening caufe of their delirious effect: However probable the contrary opinion may ftill appear to thofe, who confider that fpafm never fails to precede or to accompany the nervous diforders fubfequent to fuch application, and moreover that fpafm is fufficient to produce maniacal fymptoms; neverthelefs the neareft known caufe of Madnefs remains exactly the fame, and thefe external objects are ftill to be reckoned among its remoter caufes, which ever opinion is the more probable. Since it is impoffible for any one of them to act at all upon the nerves without motion impulfe and preffure in the fame manner and order, as if they had previoufly occafioned mufcular conftriction

striction and vascular obstruction its most usual effect.

As for Tumors by Congestion ending in Madness, that is to say those loads of fluids which gradually overcharge the vessels contiguous to the nerves, and by compressing a sufficient quantity of medullary matter create delusive sensation as effectually as does inflammation or any sudden distension of the same vessels : such gradual or chronical congestions are frequently, tho' not always, an effect of a very different sort of muscular constriction, easily distinguishable from the former by its manner of invasion and continuance. For this spasmodic action of the muscular fibres is very gentle at first, and so far from alarming either the patient or his friends, that for some time it is very little attended to or even discernable. But what it wants in violence is more than made up by its obstinate duration and encrease : inasmuch as it seldom remits, and is with great difficulty relieved by art. This species therefore of spasm must likewise be added to the remoter causes of Consequential Madness.

To such constant muscular constriction, and to the gradual or chronical congestions in the brain or mesenteric viscera thereby occasioned, the

the defpairing bigot, incapable in his own apprehenfion of being pardoned by infinite mercy,
or predeftined by infinite juftice to eternal mi-
fery before he had a being, the moping lover,
the motionlefs widow or mother bereft of her
children, may at firft view be afcribed. Who
all wear *contractæ feria frontis*, and difcover the
fixed mufcular marks of paffions flower indeed
in their operation than the turbulent ftorms of
joy or anger, but which in confequence of preffure upon the nerves are as much the remoter
caufes of Madnefs, and indeed fooner or later
are as deftructive to every animal power.

The fame Tumors by Congeftion, capable
with intervening preffure of creating Confequential Madnefs, are indeed oftentimes an effect of
laxity in the overloaded veffels themfelves. But
even this weaknefs, if traced to its original, will
frequently be found owing to one of the two
aforementioned fpecies of mufcular conftriction.

To fuch vafcular laxity arifing from mufcular
fpafm may be referred the many inftances of
Madnefs occafioned by præmature, exceffive, or
unnatural Venery, by Gonorhœas ill cured with
loads of Mercury and irritating Salts, by fevers,
and other fuch like convulfive tumults. And
from hence we may account for the chimærical
dreams

dreams of infirm and fhattered Philofophers, who after having fpent many days and nights without clofing their eyes in unwearied endeavours to reconcile metaphyfical contradictions, to fquare the circle, to difcover the Longitude or grand Secret, have at laft fallen half afleep, and who by exceffive attention of body have ftrained every animal fibre, and may without a metaphor be faid to have cracked their brains.

But, altho' laxity arifing from fpafm is moft commonly the caufe of gradual obftructions ending in delufive Senfation, neverthelefs the fame delirious tumors by Congeftion, more efpecially thofe that act upon the nervous matter contained in the abdomen, are formed fometimes without laxity or any fpafmodic diforder whatever, either by excefs of eating or by defect of voluntary motion : which motion is juft as neceffary to a due propulfion of the fluids thro' the uterine and hæmorrhoidal veffels, and thro' the many and intricate ramifications of the *vena portæ*, as is the action of the heart or the refilition of the veffels themfelves. Gluttony therefore and idlenefs are both to be added to the remoter caufes of Confequential Madnefs.

To the firft is owing the meagrim of the Epicure. To the fecond, perhaps more than to a

I

ſpirit of lying, may be aſcribed the temptations of St. *Anthony* and the lazy Monks his followers, the extaſies of ſendentary and chlorotic Nuns, and their frequent converſations with Angelic miniſters of grace. Not to mention what now and then happens to the ſenior Recluſes in our Proteſtant Monaſteries at *Oxford* and *Cambridge*.

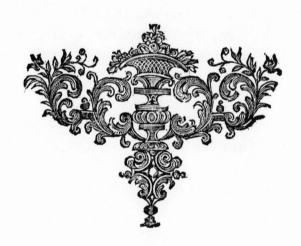

SECT.

## S E C T.   IX.

*The Diagnoftic Signs of Original and Confequen-*
*tial Madnefs ; and the Prognoftic arifing there-*
*from.*

HAVING in the two preceding Sections
difcovered moft of the caufes of Madnefs that deferve our attention, and
thereby divided this diforder into two fpecies,
*viz. Original* and *Confequential* : It will be neceffary to mention fome particular circumftances
attending either fpecies, which will enable the
Phyfician not only to diftinguifh Original Madnefs from Confequential, but alfo the better to
fettle his prognoftic and method of cure.

Firft then, there is fome reafon to fear that
Madnefs is Original, when it neither follows nor
accompanies any accident, which may juftly be
deemed its external and remoter caufe.

Secondly, there is more reafon to fear that,
whenever this diforder is hæreditary, it is Original. For, altho' even in fuch cafe it may now
and then be excited by fome external and known
caufe, yet the ftriking oddities that characterife

whole

whole families derived from Lunatic anceſtors, and the frequent breaking forth of real Madneſs in the offspring of ſuch illconcerted alliances, and that from little or no provocation, ſtrongly intimate that the nerves or inſtruments of Senſation in ſuch perſons are not originally formed perfect and like the nerves of other men.

Thirdly, we may with the greateſt degree of probability affirm that Madneſs is Original, when it both ceaſes and appears afreſh without any aſſignable cauſe. For, although we cannot gueſs why this diſeaſe of the nerves is ever relieved without the real aſſiſtance of art, or why it attacks the patient again without any new provocation, any more than we can account for the ſpontaneous intermiſſion of convulſion, fever, head-ach, and ſuch like ſpaſmodic diſorders of the muſcles ; it is however impoſſible that any one effect whatever can perfectly ceaſe, ſo long as that cauſe which was capable of producing it continues to act upon the ſame ſubject and in the ſame manner. And it is as impoſſible that the effect of any action can after a total diſcontinuance ariſe again, without its being regenerated by the ſame or at leaſt by a ſimilar action. Therefore that diſorder, be it muſcular or nervous, be it convulſion or Madneſs, which ſpontaneouſly ceaſes and as ſpontaneouſly invades

again,

again, cannot be confequential to any external caufe, which always exifts, and whofe action always continueth the fame.

Original Madnefs, whether it be hæreditary or intermitting, is not removable by any method, which the fcience of Phyfick in its prefent imperfect ftate is able to fuggeft.

But, altho' Original Madnefs is never radically cured by human art, its illconditioned fate is however a little recompenfed fometimes by a perfect recovery, fometimes by long intervals of fanity, without our affiftance and beyond our expectation. Befides Original Madnefs is in itfelf very little prejudicial to animal life. For it is notorious that men really mad live as long as thofe who are perfectly in their fenfes; and, whenever they ficken or die, they like other mortals are moft frequently attacked by illneffes, which have no neceffary connection with or dependance upon their old complaint of falfe perception.

Madnefs, which is confequential to other diforders or external caufes, altho' it now and then admits of relief by the removal or correction of fuch diforders or caufes; yet in proportion to the force and continued action of fuch caufes, and according

according to the circumftances of the preceding diforders, it is very often complicated with many other ill effects of thofe caufes and diforders; and, tho' it may not in itfelf be prejudicial to bodily health, any more than Original Madnefs, yet by its companions it becomes fatal or greatly detrimental to animal life.

Madnefs, tho' it may be Confequential at firft, frequently becomes habitual and in effect the very fame as Madnefs ftrictly Original. In which cafe the internal frame and conftitution of the nervous fubftance retains that ill difpofition which was communicated to it *ab extra*, even after that the caufe of fuch communication is quite removed or ceafes to act : And the fame fubftance, tho' formed originally as perfect as that of other men, yet by the continual and forcible action of fuch external caufe is at laft effentially vitiated in the fame manner and to as great a degree, as if it had been created imperfect and of itfelf capable of exciting delufive fenfation.

When internal exoftofes of the cranium, or induration of the Dura Mater are the caufes of Confequential Madnefs, each of thefe cafes is apparently incurable by art. Fracture or intropreffion of the cranium, and concuffion of the head, or rather its effects, tho' very dangerous and

and difficult to be managed, have fometimes been relieved.

When Infolation by the intervening rarefaction of the blood contained in the brain produces delirium, this its mifchievous effect frequently yields to the lancet, if not too late or too fparingly applied. But if Madnefs is the more immediate confequence of the Sun's action upon the nervous fubftance, and if, however occafioned it is from want of care or from obftinacy of the cafe protracted after that the piercing darts of heat its remoter caufe are quite abated, it is generally of long duration and very often incurable : forafmuch as the medullary portion of the brain is either fhocked by the continued diftenfion of the contiguous veffels, or is diftracted by the fiery impreffion in fuch a manner that its conftituent particles are quite deranged from that order, which is neceffary to the performing their natural functions in a proper manner.

Madnefs confequential to the inflammation of thofe membranes that furround the brain is very dangerous : becaufe fuch obftruction is formed in minute veffels which lie out of our reach, and which cannot be foon enough relieved by the moft plentiful evacuation ; nor can the brain thus overcharged endure any additional fhock of
errhines,

errhines, vomits, or rough purges: Since fpafm thereby excited would either endanger a rupture of the diftended veffels, or heighten the delirious preffure up to Apoplexy, or convert the inflammatory matter into mortification.

And indeed this ftate of Madnefs, called Phrenzy, let the Phyfician act ever fo fkilfully, frequently ends in one or other of the two laft mentioned cafes. The firft of which is plainly threatened by ftupidity fucceeding to delirium; and mortification of the brain may be declared coming on, or rather formed, when the maniacal fymptoms ceafe without any apparent reafon, and when the patient who was raving becomes calm and fenfible in an inftant; whilft greater debility and a pulfe hardly perceivable, together with coldnefs in the extremities, foretell that this unexpected recovery of the underftanding, however it may flatter, will be fatal.

Madnefs confequential to a gradual or chronical congeftion of fluids frequently admits of releif, if applied in time. And fuch congeftion is lefs dangerous and more eafily removed whenever the mefenteric nerves alone are thereby affected; inafmuch as every difficulty and danger that attends any injury muft be lefs the fewer thofe nerves are that fuffer the fame.

When

When fpafm is productive of obftructions upon the brain and nerves, and in this cafe becomes a-nother and a ftill remoter caufe of Confequential Madnefs, if fuch fpafm is fuddenly excited either by the tumultuous paffions of joy and anger, or by intoxicating drugs and vinous fpirits, it is indeed very violent and oftentimes fatal by its immediate effects. But in cafe the patient is ca-pable of bearing the firft fhock, and has not been weakened by frequent attacks of the fame nature; fuch fudden and irregular action of the mufcles together with all its phrenetic or mania-cal confequences is much fooner either fpontane-oufly abated or relieved by art, than the gradual and continued mufcular conftriction, which is occafioned by the more gentle paffions of love grief and defpair, or by long and uninterrupted attention to any one object however pleafing and agreeable. For Madnefs confequential to fuch obftinate mufcular conftriction muft be as obfti-nate as its caufe: and befides in this cafe of con-tinual or increafed congeftion, there is great rea-fon to fear leaft the internal frame of the nervous fubftance itfelf may at laft be effentially vitiated; and Madnefs which is habitual or of the fame nature with that which is Original may fucceed, and take the place of what at firft was only Con-fequential.

K                                         Laxity,

Laxity, whenever it intervenes between ſpaſm and delirious preſſure and thereby becomes a re-moter cauſe of Conſequential Madneſs, admits of cure if timely and properly applied; and very often the weakened membranes ſpontaneouſly re-cover their former elaſtic tone, provided the ſpaſ-modic impulſe is abated, before their conſtituent fibres are diſtracted beyond that natural tendency to approximation which was originally implanted in them.

Madneſs conſequential to gradual or chronical congeſtions occaſioned by gluttony or idleneſs eaſily yields to medical care, if ſeaſonably and properly applied.

Madneſs conſequential to or accompanied with other diſorders affords no particular prognoſtic, but what ariſes from thoſe diſorders when con-ſidered as primary diſtempers diſtinct and ſepa-rate from Madneſs itſelf.

Anxiety, when it ariſes from ſome fault in-hæring in the internal frame and conſtitution of the nervous ſubſtance, which is thereby rendered too ſenſible, like Original Madneſs and for the ſame reaſon is not radically curable. But when its only cauſe is a laxity or defect of thoſe exter-nal

nal integuments which were given to the nervous fubftance for its defence, in fuch cafe Anxiety however afflicting promifes better fuccefs.

Infenfibility or Ideotifm, when it arifes from an internal and conftitutional defect of the organs defigned to excite fenfation, or when it is a fymptom or confequence of Original Madnefs, like Original Madnefs and for the fame reafon muft be pronounced incurable by art. But, what is very remarkable and much to be lamented, when Infenfibility is the effect of Confequential Madnefs, or when it may be attributed to the præternatural clofenefs and rigidity of the nervous integuments, or to obftructions in the contiguous veffels ; tho' it may feem as curable as Confequential Anxiety, yet in fact (whatever is the reafon of the difference) it is very feldom relieved either by art or Nature.

SECT.

## SECT. X.

### *The Regimen and Cure of Madnefs.*

THE Regimen in this is perhaps of more importance than in any diftemper. It was the faying of a very eminent practitioner in fuch cafes *that management did much more than medicine*; and repeated experience has convinced me that confinement alone is oftentimes fufficient, but always fo neceffary, that without it every method hitherto devifed for the cure of Madnefs would be ineffectual.

Madnefs then, confidered as delufive Senfation unconnected with any other fymptom, requires the patient's being removed from all objects that act forcibly upon the nerves, and excite too lively a perception of things, more efpecially from fuch objects as are the known caufes of his diforder; for the fame reafon as reft is recommended to bodies fatigued, and the not attempting to walk when the ancles are ftrained.

The vifits therefore of affecting friends as well as enemies, and the impertinent curiofity of thofe, who think it paftime to converfe with Madmen

and

and to play upon their paſſions, ought ſtrictly
to be forbidden.

On the ſame account the place of confinement ſhould be at ſome diſtance from home:
and, let him be where he will, none of his own
ſervants ſhould be ſuffered to wait upon him.
For all perſons, whom he may think he hath his
accuſtomed right to command, if they diſobey
his extravagant orders will probably ruffle him
to the higheſt pitch of fury, or if they comply
will ſuffer him to continue in a diſtracted and ir-
reſolute ſtate of mind, and will leave him to the
mercy of various paſſions, any one of which
when unreſtrained is oftentimes more than ſufficient to hurry a ſober man out of his ſenſes.

Every unruly appetite muſt be checked, every
fixed imagination muſt if poſſible be diverted.
The patient's body and place of reſidence is care-
fully to be kept clean: the air he breaths ſhould
be dry and free from noiſom ſteams: his food
eaſy of digeſtion and ſimple, neither ſpirituous,
nor high ſeaſoned and full of poignancy: his
amuſements not too engaging nor too long continued, but rendered more agreeable by a well
timed variety. Laſtly his employment ſhould
be about ſuch things as are rather indifferent,
and which approach the neareſt to an intermediate

diate ſtate (if ſuch there be) between pleaſure and anxiety.

As to the cure of Madneſs, this like the cure of any other diſeaſe conſiſts, 1. In removing or correcting its cauſes : 2. In removing or correcting its ſymptoms : 3. In preventing, removing, or correcting its ill effects.

Theſe three intentions are to be anſwered either by general and rational ſcience; or, if that is wanting, by particular experience alone collected from plain and ſimilar facts, which the hiſtory of practice ſupplies us with.

Original Madneſs indeed deſerves our firſt attention, as it is the leaſt complicated with any other diſorder. But a very little reflection will ſerve to convince that all our conſideration will never enable us to treat this firſt ſpecies of Madneſs in a rational manner. For it is impoſſible by any thing like judgment or previous deſign to anſwer the firſt intention, *viz. to remove the immediate neceſſary and ſufficient cauſe of Madneſs*, which cauſe lies out of the reach even of our imagination : And, ſince no quality whatever can be corrected but by its contrary quality, therefore the unknown ſtate of the nervous ſubſtance, when exciting deluſive ſenſation, prevents

our

our applying to it any remedy, whose apparent qualities betray a manifest contrariety to such distempered state.

And as to the second and third intentions, they in Original Madness are as little to be answered as the first. But that is not because either the symptoms or the ill effects of Original Madness lye out of our reach, or their causes are unknown; but because Original Madness when considered *per se* is not accompanied with any symptoms or succeeded by any effects, which if not prevented removed or corrected would endanger the life or health of the patient.

Nor does experience, which oftentimes supplies the defect of rational intention in many disorders that are hitherto inexplicable by general science and the common laws of Nature, furnish us with any well attested remedy for Original Madness. For, altho' several specifick Medicines have by the merciful direction of Providence been of late successfully applied in some distempers otherwise incurable by art, such as Mercury in the Venereal infection, Opium in pain and watchfulness, the Peruvian Bark in mortification intermittent fevers and many other complaints; and altho' we may have reason to hope that the peculiar antidote of Madness is reserved in Nature's ture's ftore, and will be brought to light in its appointed time ; yet fuch is our prefent misfortune, that either this important fecret hath been by its inventors withheld from the reft of mankind, or, which is more probable, hath never yet been difcovered.

Since therefore the firft fpecies of Madnefs is incurable by any remedy which reafon or experience fuggefts, let us divert our attention to the fecond fpecies : And here to our great comfort we fhall find that Confequential Madnefs is frequently manageable by human art.

For, altho' delufive Senfation, by whatever external accident it may be occafioned, when confidered as a diftempered ftate of the nerves themfelves, admits of no rational or fpecific relief any more than Madnefs which is not confequential to any known caufe ; neverthelefs the previous diforders and external caufes of delufive Senfation are frequently within our reach. And this, as well as any other morbid effect, may in reafon be and in fact often is prevented or abated ; provided the known caufe is taken care of in time, that is before its continued action hath altered the nervous fubftance to fuch a degree as to have rendered it effentially or habitually unfound.

Now,

Now, forafmuch as preffure of the nervous or medullary fubftance amongft all the known and external caufes of Confequential Madnefs appears the neareft to its delirious effect, and indeed fo neceffary a caufe, that without its intervention nothing external can be fuppofed capable of exciting delufive Senfation, this caufe therefore muft be the firft object of our care.

In the next place our endeavours are to be employed in preventing removing or weakning thofe other external accidents before enumerated, which by occafioning intermediate preffure are the remoter caufes of Confequential Madnefs.

Delirious preffure of the brain or medullary fubftance contained in the nerves, which is the neareft of all the known caufes of Madnefs and therefore demands our firft attention, is incapable of being effectually relieved, except the compreffing matter itfelf be leffened, diverted, or diflodged from the part affected : or, to fpeak technically, the chief intentions under this firft article are 1. Depletion ; 2. Revulfion ; 3. Removal ; 4. Expulfion.

Not that all thefe intentions are to be anfwered in all cafes and circumftances of delirious

L                                preffure.

preſſure. For when internal exoſtoſes, induration of the Dura Mater, fracture intropreſſion
and concuſſion of the head occaſion ſuch pref-
ſure, Removal (which indeed intropreſſion does
now and then admit) is apparently impracticable.
Nor can Expulſion in any one of theſe caſes, or
indeed in any oppreſſion of the brain that is ſimilar to tumor by Fluxion, be attempted without
imminent danger to the patient's life.

But the two firſt intentions are almoſt always
to be purſued ; and delirious preſſure of the brain
or medullary ſubſtance contained in the nerves
demand Depletion and Revulſion, let its remoter
cauſes or circumſtances be what they will. For,
tho' neither of theſe intentions propoſe the removal of exoſtoſes or any one accident juſt now mentioned, yet unloading the veſſels contiguous to
the brain or nerves, which are thereby aggrieved,
will certainly in all caſes prevent or leſſen the delirious effect. And, if the preſſure ariſes ſolely
from the diſtenſion of the veſſels themſelves, Depletion and Revulſion are apparently the appoſite
and neceſſary methods of relief.

When preſſure of the brain or nerves is ſudden,
both theſe intentions may ſafely and effectually
be anſwered by the lancet and cupping-glaſs again
and again repeated in proportion to the ſtrength
of

of the patient and the greatneſs of the preſſure;
by neutral ſalts, which gently ſtimulating the in-
teſtines and ſenſible parts contained in the abdomen provoke ſtools and urine: of this ſort are
Nitre, Sal Catharticus amarus, Magneſia alba,
Tartar, and all its preparations, more eſpecially
the Sal Diureticus deſervedly recommended by
Dr. *Mead* in Maniacal caſes. And Revulſion in
particular may be ſucceſsfully attempted by the
oily and penetrating ſteams ariſing from ſkins and
other ſoft parts of animals newly ſlain, by tepid
fomentations and cataplaſms applied to the head
legs and feet, by oily and emollient glyſters;
which are of very great ſervice not only as they
empty the belly, but alſo and indeed chiefly becauſe they ſerve as a fomentation to the inteſtinal
tube, and by relaxing the branches of the aorta
deſcendens, which are here diſtributed in great
number, make it more capable of receiving the
blood; which will therefore according to the
known courſe of fluid matter be diverted from
the head.

The ſame intentions of Depletion and Revulſion ſeem indeed to recommend ſinapiſms, cau-
ſtics, errhines, and veſicatories, as alſo the
rougher cathartics, emetics, and volatile diaphoretics. But when we reflect that a ſpaſmodic
conſtriction is by no means the leaſt amongſt the

remoter

remoter caufes of Madnefs, we fhall in every cafe of fudden preffure be fearful of any powerful irritation that endangers conftriction, and that cannot anfwer either intention unlefs it previoufly excites an irregular action of the mufcles.

And indeed Phrenfy or fudden preffure of the brain attended with inflammation of the containing membranes, and intrufion of blood and ferum into improper veffels of the head, not only forbid finapifms and every powerful irritation, but incline us to be fufpicious of cathartic falts in too large dofes, and even of Nitre itfelf, tho' it is reckoned fpecifically antiphlogiftic, and tho' it is fuccefsfully adminiftered in many other inflammatory tumors before they fuppurate.

Delirious Preffure of the nervous fubftance contained either in the head or abdomen, when gradual or chronical, tho' it is of a very different nature from fudden preffure, and tho' it is fimilar to tumor by Congeftion, yet in robuft and plethoric habits alike indicates Depletion and Revulfion. But, if the fubject is either naturally infirm or fhattered and exhaufted by preceding illnefs, the lancet muft be cautioufly ufed or entirely forbidden ; and both thefe intentions can with fafety be anfwered by nothing except the mildeft folutives, fuch as the neutral falts above-
mentioned,

mentioned, Caſſia, Manna, &c. and the Gumms quickened with a few grains of Aloes.

But, when delirious preſſure of the nervous ſub-ſtance, more particularly that contained in the abdomen, is gradual or chronical, if ſuch gentle evacuants, tho' often and properly repeated, prove unable to leſſen or relieve the ſtagnating matter, and in caſe the weakneſs of the patient does not contraindicate, here the third and fourth intentions take place: and it becomes abſolutely neceſſary to ſhake with violence the head and hypochondria by convulſing the muſcular fibres with emetics rougher purges and errhines. For ſuch ſpaſmodic action communicates a vibrating motion to the ſolid fibres of the whole body; whereby the overloaded membranes and integu-ments that compreſs the contiguous medullary ſubſtance remove or expell their morbid contents, and the patient delivered from his delirious in-cumbrances frequently recovers his former ſanity of mind as well as body.

SECT.

## SECT. XI.

### *The Cure of Madness.*

PRessure of the medullary matter contained in the brain and nerves, amongst all the known causes of Madness the nearest to such its delirious effect, and therefore the first object of our attention, has been considered with regard to such methods of cure as are indicated by reason and justifyed by experience. In the next place therefore we are to turn our thoughts to those *other external accidents, which by occasioning intermediate pressure are the remoter causes of Consequential Madness.*

Now the several remoter causes before enumerated, were 1. Internal exostoses of the cranium; 2. Induration of the Dura Mater; 3. Fracture or intropression of the skull and concussion of the head; 4. Insolation; 5. One species of spasm, or muscular constriction, sudden and impetuous but sooner quieted; which arises either from 6. Material objects external to the body, *viz.* poisons, medicines, and vinous spirits, or from 7. Tumultuous passions, *viz.* joy and anger; 8. Another species of spasm or muscular

con-

conftriction more gradual and gentle in its attack,
but frequently encreafing, and almoft always obftinate in its duration; which arifes from 9. Unwearied attention of the mind to one object, or
from the quieter paffions of love, grief, or defpair;
10. Præternatural laxity of the membranes or veffels contiguous to the nerves; 11. Gluttony; 12.
Idlenefs. Of all which in their order.

*Internal exoftofes and induration of the Dura
Mater* cannot be prevented, nor does either cafe
admit of any particular method of relief. *Concuffion* may itfelf indeed be fometimes prevented,
but its ill effects can never be prevented or removed by any intention except that of Depletion
and Revulfion recommended under the firft article of cure. In *fracture or intropreffion of the
fkull* the trepan is peculiarly adapted either to
give a vent to, or to remove the extravafated and
ftagnating fluids.

*Infolation* is quite out of our power; but its
fubject we have to deal with is not always fo.
For, altho' the fiery darts of heat are not capable
of being removed or leffened by human means,
the patient may be removed; or, when that cannot eafily be done, the head may be fecured by
a proper integument; for which purpofe a cap

of

of thick paper has been fuccefsfully recommended.

*Spafm* or mufcular conftriction, as well the
fudden and impetuous as the more gradual and
gentle, when confidered by its felf and as ab-
ftracted from irritation or any external caufe, admits of no method of cure fuggefted by rational
intention : Forafmuch as the immediate neceffary and fufficient caufe of mufcular action, be it
natural or diftempered, is abfolutely unknown.
Whenever therefore nothing external to the mufcular fibres can be affigned which is capable of
provoking their conftriction, we have no hope
except in fpecific remedies, that is in fuch drugs,
whofe antifpafmodic virtues experience alone has
difcovered.

Under this head of antifpafmodics every one,
I fuppofe, will readily place Valerian, Caftor, the
Gumms, and Mufk ; and, were I at liberty to in-
dulge a fufpicion which has for fome time oc-
curred, I fhould be inclined to add Nitre, the
Magnefia, the Sal Diureticus, as alfo all alcaline
fubftances incorporated with acids, all neutral
falts, and all alexipharmacs or diaphoretics : whofe
fudden efficacy in appeafing the paroxyfms of
feverifh diforders which are apparently fpafmodic can be attributed to no other known power,
but

but such as hath an immediate influence upon the animal fibres endued with motion. Not that any thing more than conjecture is hereby proposed; which is to be admitted or not, as the conclusions of others arising from their own just reasoning and experience shall determine.

But, whatever class the virtues of Nitre and neutral salts &c. shall hereafter be ranked under, it may at present with great truth be asserted from observations already made that they are the only specific helps, which can be depended on with any probability of success or even with safety in fits of Madness attended with fury and violent spasmodic motions. And it is as certain that those other anti-spasmodic drugs which are poinant and irritating, *viz.* Valerian, Castor, and the gumms, are serviceable and indeed harmless only in the second or gradual and gentler species of muscular constriction.

Which observations by the way not only serve to distinguish what specific remedies are proper for either case of spasmodic Madness; but moreover suggest a caution to the Physician in the administring even Nitre and other saline febrifuges in spasmodic disorders whether delirious or not: because such sharp bodies when over-dosed or when applied to subjects too susceptible of irrita-

M                                                        tion

tion may fometimes aggravate every fymptom they are intended to relieve, and may become as mifchievous as thofe other more poinant anti-fpafmodics have frequently proved, when pre-fcribed in all convulfive cafes under the general and improper title of *Nervous Medicines*.

The fame caution is likewife highly neceffary when fpafm is occafioned by the fixth clafs of re-moter caufes, *viz. poifons, medicines, vinous fpi-rits*, or any affignable matter which actually excites an irregular motion of the mufcles. For it is almoft felf-evident that in fuch cafe all addi-tional irritation muft increafe every convulfive effect, and that even the moft gentle faline re-medies will be hazardous or at beft inefficacious, until the material caufe of fpafm if fuperficial is removed by chirurgical affiftance, if it be in the ftomach or inteftines until it is difcharged by the force of vomits or purges, or if fuch means of expulfion be thought too violent until the offending matter is fufficiently enervated by di-luting and abforbing medicines, or in cafe of ex-tream neceffity until its effect is prevented or ftifled by narcotics. All which different methods of cure in fuch Confequential Madnefs muft be left to the fagacity of the Phyfician; it being im-poffible to lay down any general direction in a

matter

matter attended with fo great a variety of unfore-
feen accidents.

But, though the removal of the fixth clafs of
remoter caufes, *viz.* every irritation which produces Madnefs, is not always feafible or even fafe,
and though fuch terrible effect admits of no relief fo long as the material caufe continues to act,
neverthelefs prevention, at leaft with regard to
vinous fpirits, is entirely in our power. For which
reafon it deferves the ferious confideration of our
governors, how far it is their duty by a total prohi-
bition of the caufe to prevent thofe frequent
effects of temporary but real Lunacy, for which
many wretches are executed, who in reality
are guilty of debauchery alone, which has been
rendered familiar by the cuftom or rather the
convenience of their country, and is allowed or
commuted for by the laws of the revenue.

As to the feventh clafs of remoter caufes, *viz.*
*tumultuous and fpafmodic paffions, fuch as joy and*
*anger,* in cafe the patient is not in immediate
danger of his life, nothing of any great confequence is to be done at firft ; in hopes that thefe
paffions and their mufcular effects will, as they
are frequently known to do, fubfide of themfelves. But, whenever *anceps remedium* is the indi-
cation, after fufficient depletion and diminution

of

of maniacal preſſure thereby occaſioned, we muſt have recourſe to the ſpecific, that is to the unaccountably narcotic virtues of the Poppy. And, if notwithſtanding this temporary relief any one particular paſſion ſeems to engroſs the man or continues beyond its uſual period, in ſuch caſe the diſcretion of the Phyſician muſt determine how far it may be adviſeable or ſafe to ſtifle it by a contrary paſſion. I ſay _ſafe_, becauſe it is almoſt impoſſible by general reaſoning to foretell what will be the effect of fear ſubſtituted in the room of anger, or of ſorrow immediately ſucceeding to joy.

The eighth remoter cauſe of Conſequential Madneſs, _viz. Muſcular Conſtriction, gradual, gentler and uniform, but more obſtinate_, may ſometimes be relieved or as it were diverted by convulſion that is by an alternate motion of muſcular fibres artificially excited in ſome other part of the body. On which account veſicatories, vomits, rough cathartics, errhines, and the moſt poinant amongſt the medicines called nervous, may in this particular caſe of ſpaſm become even antiſpaſmodic. For, ignorant as we are and perhaps ſhall always be of the reaſon, experience has ſhewn that, although many parts of the body may be convulſed together, one ſpecies of ſpaſm

however

however occafioned feldom fails to put an end to that other which before fubfifted.

When the ninth clafs of remoter caufes demands our care, *viz. unwearied attention to any one object*, as alfo *love, grief, and defpair*; any of thefe affections will fometimes be annihilated by the tumultuous but lefs dangerous and fooner fubfiding paffions of anger or joy. But, if fuch inftantaneous alteration from one extreme to the other appears either not feafible or too fhocking to be attempted with fafety; bodily pain may be excited to as good a purpofe and without any the leaft danger. It being a known obfervation, though as much out of the reach of human reafon as are moft others which occur in the animal œconomy, that no two different perceptions can fubfift at the fame time any more than the two different fpecies of morbid mufcular action, *viz. the convulfive and the conftrictive*. Therefore veficatories, cauftics, vomits, rough cathartics, and errhines, may be and in fact often are as ferviceable in this cafe of fixed nervous Senfation as in obftinate mufcular conftriction, inafmuch as they all relieve and divert the mind from its delirious attention, or from the bewitching paffions of love, grief, and defpair.

The

The tenth remoter cauſe of Conſequential Madneſs, *viz. Laxity* of thoſe veſſels or membranes that are contiguous to the nervous ſubſtance, apparently indicates ſuch remedies as have the experienced though unaccountable efficacy of contracting the material particles which conſtitute an animal body. Of this nature is iron, vitriol, and mineral waters impraegnated therewith : but above all, when nothing contraindicates, the bathing in cold or rather ſea-water.

As to the eleventh and twelfth remoter cauſes, *viz. Gluttony* and *Idleneſs,* little is requiſite for their particular cure : ſince, after proper evacuations, temperance is undoubtedly the appoſite remedy of the one, and bodily exerciſe of the other. Both which means of preſent recovery and of prevention for the future may be effectually preſcribed to men of either character, at leaſt whilſt they are actually mad and properly confined. For the diet of the glutton in ſuch caſe is abſolutely in the Phyſician's power. And, although it would be no eaſy taſk to perſwade or even to force any perſon, whether a Lunatic or not, who has long indulged in idleneſs, to put his body in motion ; nevertheleſs this ſtate of inactivity may be artificially broke through by vomits, rough cathartics, errhines, or any other
irritating

irritating medicines : which in this cafe therefore
anfwer more than one intention, and not only
difcharge or diflodge the delirious load of ftagnating fluids, but alfo by their convulfive influence
upon the mufcles of the abdomen and indeed
upon every animal fibre of the agitated body
crowd as it were a great deal of exercife into a
fmall portion of time, and that without the con-
fent of the patient, or even the trouble of con-
tradicting his lazy inclinations.

SECT.

## SECT. XII.

*The cure of the symptoms and consequences of Madness. And some observations upon the whole.*

IT may be recollected that the cure of Madness, as well as of all other distempers, consists in 1. Removing or correcting its causes: 2. Removing or correcting its symptoms: 3. Preventing, removing, or correcting its ill effects.

A method of answering the first intention has been proposed in the two foregoing Sections : the symptoms and ill effects of Madness should therefore be our next care.

But Original Madness, as hath been before observed, is not necessarily accompanied with any symptoms or succeeded by any effects, that are strictly speaking insalubrious.

And indeed, with respect to Consequential Madness, whatever may accompany it as a symptom or follow it as a seeming effect, every such accidental disorder hath in reality no necessary connection with Madness itself : but is either re-

solveable

folveable into other injuries quite foreign to Maniacal affections; or, if it is owing to any one remoter caufe of Madnefs, it is ftill no more than another effect of the fame caufe; which effect is juft as capable of being thereby generated, whether Madnefs is or is not produced together with fuch fymptom or before fuch confequence.

For which reafon every fymptom and every feeming ill effect of Madnefs, whether Original or Confequential, muft be confidered either as a primary diftemper, or as the effect of fome primary diftemper, to which a proper method of cure is applicable feparate and independent of Madnefs; and therefore it is not the fubject of our prefent enquiry.

But, as Anxiety frequently precedes Madnefs like its caufe or accompanies it like its fymptom, and as Infenfibility fometimes fucceeds Madnefs like its effect; tho' both thefe præternatural ftates of Senfation are as diftinguifhable and actually feparate from delufive fenfation, as any other animal diftemper is or can well be: the fame reafons however, which required a more particular enquiry into the nature and origin of thefe two nervous affections, will excufe our endeavouring to inveftigate what method of cure the

N                                    difcovery

difcovery of their caufes may feem to indicate with any the leaft probability of fuccefs.

Anxiety then is either Original or Confequential. For, as hath been before obferved, it may arife, 1. From fome ill-conditioned ftate of the internal and proper fubftance of the nerves affected; 2. From the intolerable impulfe of external objects, or from fome defect in thofe integuments and membranes that furround the medullary matter, and when they are perfect defend it even from the natural action of bodies which would otherwife excite too lively a fenfation.

Anxiety, when it is Original, refembles Original Madnefs, and for the fame reafon feems as much out of the reach of medical affiftance: But in fact its cafe is more fortunate; and, tho' Original Anxiety is juft as incapable as Original Madnefs of being relieved by rational intention, it is however frequently palliated by more than one fpecific remedy.

For wine, and even vinous fpirits which are rightly forbidden to perfons in perfect health, when occafionally adminiftered as medicines to animal bodies agonifing with exquifite fenfation, beguile the diftreffes of mortals, and oftentimes

procure

procure them tranquillity and happiness, to which they have long been strangers. And, altho' neither wine nor vinous spirits are adviseable in the vexatious symptom of watchfulness, which frequently attends upon Anxiety, whether accompanied by Madness or not; forasmuch as such poinant stimuli must irritate before their narcotic virtues can take effect; yet I have often prescribed the *Extractum Thebaicum* from one to five grains without any ill consequence to such mad patients as were uneasy and raving all the night as well as day. And, where extream weakness or some approaches to stupor rendered this powerful narcotic not quite so safe, Camphire and Sagapenum have afforded the same anodyne and soporific virtues, tho' not to so great a degree.

Nor ought any one to reject such temporary expedients, as unworthy the attention of a Physician in Original Anxiety, even tho' it should prove incurable by art; who considers that it is his duty to protract the misery of his fellow-creatures, if it be but for a moment; and that anodynes are absolutely necessary in every case of Consequential Anxiety, untill either the intolerable impulse of external objects can be entirely removed or weakened by such methods as particular circumstances require, or untill the

nervous

nervous integuments can be reftored to their natural firmnefs by the aftringent virtues of the Peruvian Bark, iron, vitriol, mineral waters, and cold bathing; which are the proper and oftentimes effectual remedies, whenever Anxiety arifes from the laxity or defect of thofe membranes that furround and defend the medullary matter.

Infenfibility, Idiotifm, Folly, or whatever name it is ufually known by, is, as hath been obferved, almoft always beyond the power of rational or fpecific relief. Neverthelefs, that nothing may be left untried, it feems advifeable to make general evacuations, and to contrive partial but conftant difcharges of the fluids from the head and neck by perpetual blifters, fetons, and iffues. It may likewife be of fome fervice, if nothing contraindicates, to fhake the whole folid frame by vomits, cathartics, errhines, and all forts of tolerable irritation. To which may be added, but not without great caution, the fubtle and penetrating particles contained in mineral waters drank at the fountain-head, and the concuffive force of the cold-bath or fea-water.

But if Infenfibility is conftitutional, or owing to the firm and healthy ftructure of thofe folid
                                                    membranes

membranes which sheath the nervous matter, such natural defect or impediment is incurable by art. However this state of stupidity may, at least by those who are endued with too lively a sensation, be deemed a kind of negative happiness, and rather to be envied than lamented.

And thus ends our inquiry into the causes effects and cure of Madness. But, before we quit this subject, it may not be improper to subjoin a few remarks, which will readily occur to every one who recollects the premisses, and is moreover satisfied of their reasonableness.

We have therefore, as Men, the pleasure to find that Madness is, contrary to the opinion of some unthinking persons, as manageable as many other distempers, which are equally dreadful and obstinate, and yet are not looked upon as incurable : and that such unhappy objects ought by no means to be abandoned, much less shut up in loathsome prisons as criminals or nusances to the society.

We are likewise, as Physicians, taught a very useful lesson, *viz.* That, altho' Madness is frequently
quently

quently taken for one fpecies of diforder, neverthelefs, when thoroughly examined, it difcovers
as much variety with refpect to its caufes and
circumftances as any diftemper whatever : Madnefs therefore, like moft other morbid cafes,
rejects all general methods, *v. g.* bleeding, blifters, cauftics, rough cathartics, the gumms and
fætid antihyfterics, opium, mineral waters, cold
bathing, and vomits.

For bleeding, tho' apparently ferviceable and
neceffary in inflammation of the brain, in rarefaction of the fluids, or a plethoric habit of body, is however no more the adequate and conftant cure of Madnefs, than it is of fever. Nor
is the lancet, when applied to a feeble and con-
vulfed Lunatic, lefs deftructive than a fword.

And, altho' blifters, cauftics, and fharp purges quickned with white Hellebore, and indeed
all painful applications, not only evacuate and
thereby relieve delirious preffure, but alfo roufe
and exercife the body, and feem more peculiarly adapted to Infenfibility when it is a fymptom
or confequence of Madnefs ; neverthelefs thefe
and all pungent fubftances are to be tried with
great caution, or rather are not to be tried at
all in fits of fury. Nor does even defect of
fenfation allow their ufe, whenever fuch defect is
occafioned

occafioned by the preceding excefs of the nervous energy, or when it is accompanied with fpafm. As to black Hellebore, it is either not the drug which was recommended by the Antients and made *Anticyra* famous, or elfe it did not really deferve fuch recommendation. For after feveral trials I have not the leaft reafon to think it of any fervice in Madnefs.

For the fame reafon the gumms and all fœtid antihyfterics, which are undoubtedly ferviceable in Madnefs arifing from or complicated with fome forts of fpafmodic diforders, are by no means even fafe in all præternatural actions of the mufcles : much lefs can fuch irritating objects be proper in that particular cafe of Madnefs which is attended with feaverifh heat, which happens in a plethoric habit of body, or which follows an inflammatory obftruction in the brain.

As to Opium, notwithftanding what hath been before faid concerning the great relief obtained by this powerful drug in fome particular circumftances, it is no more a fpecific in Madnefs than it is in the Small Pox. For no good whatever can be expected but from its narcotic virtue, and much harm may arife therefrom when improperly adminiftered. For it is almoft felf-evident that in Madnefs attended with de-

bility

bility and languor, or which approaches towards
ftupor and infenfibility, every thing that deadens
fenfation muft be highly detrimental when given
in a fufficient quantity, and may prove fatal
when overdofed.

Mineral waters drank at the fountain head and
bathing in the fea or cold frefh water have been
fometimes chiefly if not folely relied on in the
cure of Madnefs, more efpecially when attended
with Anxiety and known by the name of Melancholy. Neverthelefs fuch methods of relief
are all apparently contraindicated, whenever there
is fufficient reafon to fufpect that irrefoluble congeftions of the fluids clog the membranes contiguous to the nervous fubftance, or that the folids are ftrained beyond the poffibility of recover-
ing their natural elafticity. For in cafe of irrefoluble congeftions every drop of water, whether mineral or not, taken into the circulation
will be added to the obftructing matter ; and
the contracting force of cold or of fea-water applied externally will make the fame matter more
incapable, if poffible, of being refolved. And,
when the folids are irrecoverably ftrained, they
will be in great danger of rupture or at leaft of
a farther difunion of their conftituent particles
by the expanfive force of mineral fprings, as well
as by the rude fhock of cold or of fea-water,
which

which is very senfibly felt even by thofe bodies, whofe folids are ftrong enough to bear the fame without being hurt thereby.

Laftly with refpect to Vomits, tho' it may feem almoft hæretical to impeach their antimaniacal virtues; yet, when we reflect that the good effects which can be rationally propofed from fuch fhocking operations are all neverthelefs the confequences of a morbid convulfion, thefe active medicines are apparently contraindicated, whenever there is reafon to fufpect that the veffels of the brain or nervous integuments are fo much clogged or ftrained as to endanger a rupture or further difunion, inftead of a deliverance from their oppreffive loads. The fame objection equally holds good againft fuch mufcular irritation, whenever the veffels are contracted with exceffive cold, or when their contents are rarefied by heat, as alfo in conftitutions that are lax and feeble or naturally fpafmodic, and in feveral other circumftances which need no particular defcription.

Befides, fince the characters that diftinguifh Original from Confequential Madnefs are not always fo clear and certain as to leave no room for error, and fince Original Madnefs is not curable by any method which human reafon or ex-

O                                    perience

perience hath hitherto been able to difcover ; we
fhould take great care not to do harm where it
is not in our power to do any good, and not
dwell too long on endeavouring to remove the
caufes of Madnefs, which perhaps are only imaginary, more efpecially if the methods to be
made ufe of are by no means indifferent. For
which reafon, whenever upon fufficient tryal not
only of vomits but even of rougher purges, tho'
rationally indicated at firft, the patient grows
worfe or at leaft gains no ground, they are all
entirely to be laid afide. For, if in any cafe the
*juvantia* and *lædentia* fupply us with medical
knowledge, they moft fignally do fo in diforders,
whofe nature we are not thoroughly acquainted
with, and where reafoning *a priori* cannot certainly foretell the fuccefs of any one application.

Nor let us immediately defpair at being obliged to withhold that affiftance which feemed the
moft effectual, or conclude that, becaufe the
patient cannot be relieved by art, he therefore
cannot be relieved at all. For Madnefs, like feveral other animal diftempers, oftentimes ceafes
fpontaneoufly, that is without our being able to
affign a fufficient reafon ; and many a Lunatic,
who by the repetition of vomits and other convulfive ftimuli would have been ftrained into
downright

downright Idiotifm, has when given over as incurable recovered his underftanding.

To which remarks arifing as juft conclufions
from reafoning upon the unavoidable action of
vomits and rougher purges, I fhall beg leave to
add fome cautions, which experience has fuggefted as neceffary to be communicated to the
young practitioner, even when fuch active medicines are proper. *viz.* 1. If the feafon of the
year is in the choice of the Phyfician, to prefer
the Spring or Autumn, as being in neither extream
of cold or heat : 2. Not to perfift in their ufe at
any one time for a longer term than fix or eight
weeks : 3. Even during that term to give a re-
fpite every other or at leaft every third week from
all drugs except the gumms, neutral falts, or gentle folutives : 4. As foon as the patient vifibly
approaches to a ftate of fanity, entirely to dif-
continue thefe and all other violent methods ;
that the animal fibres, which have been ftrained
either by the caufes of Madnefs or perhaps by
the means of removing them, may be at liberty to recover their natural firmnefs and juft
approximation of particles, which a repeated
concuffion will certainly prevent.

*F    I    N    I    S.*